AF430879

Textbook of
Pharmacovigilance
Concept and Practice
Second Edition

Textbook of Pharmacovigilance
Concept and Practice
Second Edition

Guru Prasad Mohanta

M. Pharm., Ph. D.

Professor and Head

Prabal Kumar Manna

M . Pharm., Ph. D.

Professor and Former Head,
Department of Pharmacy,
Annamalai University,
Annamalai Nagar – 608 002.

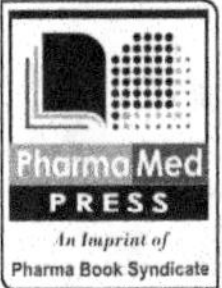

PharmaMed Press

An imprint of Pharma Book Syndicate

A unit of BSP Books Pvt. Ltd.

4-4-309/316, Giriraj Lane,
Sultan Bazar, Hyderabad - 500 095.

Textbook of Pharmacovigilance: *Concept and Practice, Second Edition*
by Guru Prasad Mohanta and Prabal Kumar Manna

© 2021, 2016, *by Authors and Publisher*

Disclaimer: The authors and the publishers have taken due care to provide the authentic, reliable and up to date information related to the subject. However, neither the authors nor the publisher shall be responsible for any liability for any damage caused as a result of use of this book. The respective user must check the accuracy from other sources too.

Published by

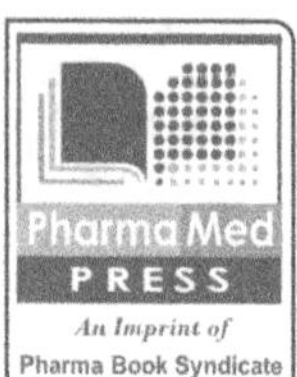

PharmaMed Press
An imprint of Pharma Book Syndicate

A unit of BSP Books Pvt. Ltd.
4-4-309/316, Giriraj Lane, Sultan Bazar, Hyderabad - 500 095.
Phone: 040-23445600, 23445688; Fax: 91+40-23445611
E-mail: info@pharmamedpress.com
www.pharmamedpress.com/pharmamedpress.net

ISBN: 978-93-89974-13-3

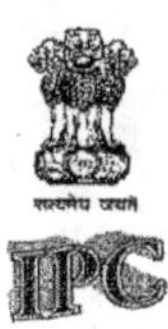

INDIAN PHARMACOPOEIA COMMISSION
National Coordination Centre, Pharmacovigilance Programme of India
MINISTRY OF HEALTH & FAMILY WELFARE, GOVERNMENT OF INDIA
SECTOR-23, RAJ NAGAR, GHAZIABAD- 201 002.

Tel No: 0120- 6582849, 2783392, 2783400, 2783401; Fax: 2783311
Mail: pvpi@ipcindia.net, Web: www.ipc.gov.in

FOREWORD

Pharmacovigilance has been accepted as an important public health function which aims at reducing the medicine related harms. Intensive efforts are currently ongoing in the country to strengthen the system of Pharmacovigilance Programme of India (PvPI) to ensure the safety of medicines. The PvPI involves a systematic collection of adverse drug reactions (ADRs) data and providing valuable information to drug regulatory authority to take necessary actions in order to promote patients safety.

However, lack of knowledge of where, what and how to report ADRs continue to be the major concern of PvPI. As the entire healthcare professionals are important stakeholders in Pharmacovigilance, it may be more appropriate to educate, train and sensitize them during their course itself on various aspects of Pharmacovigilance.

This book entitled "Textbook of Pharmacovigilance: *Concept and Practice*" provides a unique and valuable resource for learning as well as practicing Pharmacovigilance. I hope the healthcare students and the professionals will find this book of great use to understand the standard definitions, terminologies and other essential elements of Pharmacovigilance. The authors, Dr. Guru Prasad Mohanta and Dr. Prabal Kumar Manna, with their long experience in teaching and reasonable experience in Pharmacovigilance have put their effort in presenting the key principles of Pharmacovigilance in simple language for easy adaptability. Hope the students would find chapters on case studies and global scenario more interesting as they give insight on global activities and scope.

I do hope the book will be used as an important educational intervention tool to promote Pharmacovigilance activities both in health systems and in the industries.

V. Kalaiselvan
Principal Scientific Officer

PREFACE TO THE SECOND EDITION

Either write something worth reading or Do something worth writing.

Benjamin Franklin

The authors have great pleasure of presenting the Second Edition of Textbook of Pharmacovigilance: Concept and Practice. Pharmacovigilance is a dynamic and constantly evolving field. Its structure has changed over time from sudden crisis management to sudden drugs withdrawal to a scientific discipline in its own right. 40th year Anniversary of Safety Monitoring of Medicines was observed in early 2018 by World Health Organization and Uppsala Monitoring Centre.

In India too, there has been tremendous growth and recognition of pharmacovigilance activities. The Pharmacovigilance system has been made mandatory for marketing authorization holders to achieving the status of WHO Collaborating Centre for Pharmacovigilance in Public Health Programmes and Regulatory Services for Indian Pharmacopeia Commission, National Pharmacovigilance Coordination Centre.

The new edition has many revised and expanded chapters in addition to new chapters for Pharmacovigilance of Vaccines, Materiovigilance and Haemovigilance. While writing the texts we have given the readers' interest and pharmacovigilance activities in India as primary focus. Elaborate details of pharmacovigilance need for exporters of medicines including ICH and requirements of the need of importing countries could be missing. But this is beyond the scope of this short textbook basically intended to provide fundamental knowledge on pharmacovigilance and practice requirements in Indian context.

We would like to express our gratitude to our family members: (Reena, Anupam and Amrita of Guru Prasad Mohanta) and (Nibedita, Pratiksha and Praseed of Prabal Kumar Manna) for encouraging and allowing us to revise the text. Our publisher, Mr. Anil Shah, deserves special appreciation for timely encouragement and bringing out the text at shortest period of time.

This is our small attempt to educate the students who wish to choose pharmacovigilance as career. We are grateful to numerous readers for their encouraging feedback and we hope the second edition would also receive similar patronage.

Guru Prasad Mohanta
[gpmohanta@hotmail.com]

Prabal Kumar Manna
[prabalmanna@gmail.com]

PREFACE TO THE FIRST EDITION

"There are many who come and go
There are few who leave a mark"

Pharmacovigilance in simplest sense is to "detect the harmful effects of drugs (or medicines) on patients and to reduce the likelihood of their occurrence". This is a new young discipline in Health Sciences but gaining fast acceptance among the health professionals and medicine regulating authorities. India sets to become hub for Pharmacovigilance activities as evident from the large number of IT companies venturing into this area.

Though the subject has lot of relevance in providing quality care to the patients, perhaps there is no regular programme, other than some pharmacy programmes, where the subject is extensively taught. There are few short term courses offered by unorganised sectors. There are very few affordable books too. The authors made a modest attempt to educate and sensitize people who are interested in Pharmacovigilance. While authors are well aware of difficulties writing a textbook on this new emerging science, they are confident in effectively distilling the principles and facts into the present text.

The number, severity and cost of Adverse Drug Reactions (ADRs) have been recognised as a significant public health issue. There has been continuing interest in discovering what causes them and how their occurrences can be predicted or prevented, if feasible. These are the subject matters of the present text. The term drug and medicine have been used interchangeably in the whole text. The authors express their gratitude to the World Health Organization (WHO) for permitting to reproduce some of the materials of WHO in the text. The two chapters, Quality Assurance in Pharmacovigilance and Case Studies on Causality Assessment, are contributed by Mr. Shaikh Ruhu Al Amin and Dr. J. Ponni respectively. These two former students of ours, now successful Pharmacovigilance Professionals, deserve our special appreciation.

We hope the text would help the students and aspiring professionals to acquire the knowledge, necessary skills, and attitudes that would enable them to effectively identify, assess and report ADRs as well as initiate appropriate action besides taking up career in medicine safety programme.

We are grateful to Dr. G. N. Singh, Drugs Controller General of India, for encouragement and gesture of wishing for our effort in developing the text. He is also the Secretary – cum – Scientific Director of Indian Pharmacopoeia Commission and personality responsible for bringing the PV Programme of the Country to such an appreciable level. We are extremely thankful to Dr. V. Kalaiselvan, Principal Scientific Officer at Indian Pharmacopoeia Commission, Government of India, for writing the Foreword for the text. He is the key person coordinating the Pharmacovigilance Programme of India at the National Coordinating Centre (NCC). We appreciate our former student, Dr. Thota Prasad, currently Scientific Assistant at NCC, for extending his expertise throughout the entire period of preparing the text.

We would like to thank the Annamalai University Authorities for permitting us to write the text. We are thankful to our family members for bearing with us during the development of the text. Our PharmD student, Mr. V. Venkatesh, needs a special appreciation for drawing some figures for the book. We express our thanks to Mr. Anil Shah of Pharma Med Press for showing continued interest in publishing the book.

There is nothing more important than hearing the opinion of readers or users of the book. Your opinion matters us and would help us improving the text further to make it more useful.

"Let's act together to make the medicines safer for us and for our next generation as well".

Guru Prasad Mohanta
[gpmohanta@hotmail.com]

Prabal Kumar Manna
[prabalmanna@gmail.com]

CONTENTS

ABBREVIATIONS

ADR	–	Adverse Drug Reaction
ADRAC	–	Adverse Drug Reaction Advisory Committee
ADROIT	–	ADR Online Information Tracking
AEFI	–	Adverse Event Following Immunization
AHWP	–	Asian Harmonization Working Party
AIIA	–	All India Institute of Ayurveda
AIIMS	–	All India Institute of Medical Sciences
ANM	–	Auxiliary Nurse Midwife
APC	–	Ayurvedic Pharmacopoeia Committee
ASU	–	Ayurveda, Siddha and Unani
AYUSH	–	Ayurveda, Yoga and Naturopathy, Unani, Siddha and Homeopathy
BCPNN	–	Bayesian Confidence Propagation Neural Network
BNF	–	British National Formulary
CBER	–	Centre for Biologics Evaluation and Research
CDER	–	Centre for Drug Evaluation and Research
CDSCO	–	Central Drugs Standard Control Organization
CEM	–	Cohort Event Monitoring
CIOMS	–	Council for International Organizations of Medical Sciences
COHM/CHM	–	Commission on Human Medicines
CSD	–	Committee on Safety of Drugs
CSM	–	Committee on Safety of Medicines
CT	–	Clinical Trial
DCC	–	Drugs Consultative Committee
DCGI	–	Drugs Controller General of India
DIO	–	District Immunization Officer
DoTS	–	Dose, Time and Susceptibility

EHR	–	Electronic Health Record
EMP	–	Essential Medicines and Health Products
EU	–	European Union
EURD	–	European Union Reference Data
FAERS	–	FDA Adverse Event Reporting System
FDC	–	Food, Drug and Cosmetic
FSCA	–	Field Safety Corrective Action
GPvP	–	Good Pharmacovigilance Practice
HIS	–	Health System and Innovation
HPC	–	Homeopathic Pharmacopoeia Committee
HvP	–	Haemovigilance Programme
ICH	–	International Council for Harmonisation of Technical Requirements for Pharmaceuticals for Human Use
ICMR	–	Indian Council for Medical Research
ICSR	–	Individual Case Safety Report
IHN	–	International Haemovigilance Network
IMDRF	–	International Medical Device Regulators Forum
IPC	–	Indian Pharmacopoeia Commission
IPvCs	–	Intermediary Pharmacovigilance Centres (ASU &H Medicines)
ISM	–	Indian System of Medicine
ITSU	–	Immunization Technical Support Unit
LMICs	–	Least and Middle Income Countries
MAH	–	Marketing Authorization Holder
MCC	–	Medicines Control Council
MDAE	–	Medical Device Adverse Event
MDAERF	–	Medical Device Adverse Event Reporting Form
MDR	–	Multi Drug Resistant
MGPS	–	Multi-item Gamma Poisson Shrinker
MHRA	–	Medicine and Health Products Regulatory Agency

MMR	–	Measles, Mumps and Rubella
MRI	–	Magnetic Resonance Imaging
MvP	–	Materio Vigilance Programme [Medical Device]
MvPI	–	Materio Vigilance Programme of India
NBDVP	–	National Blood Donors Vigilance Programme
NCAR	–	National Competent Authority Report
NCC	–	National Coordination Centre
NHM	–	National Health Mission
NHSRC	–	National Health System Resource Centre
NPvC	–	National Pharmacovigilance Centre (ASU&H Medicines)
OMSM	–	Office of Medicine Safety Monitoring
P&P	–	Patent & Proprietary
PAC	–	Programme Approval Committee / Project Appraisal Committee
PADER	–	Periodic Adverse Drug Experience Report
PAER	–	Periodic Adverse Experience Report
PBRER	–	Periodic Benefit Risk Evaluation Report
PCIM&H	–	Pharmacopoeial Commission of Indian Medicine and Homeopathy
PHC	–	Primary Health Centre
PMS	–	Post Marketing Surveillance
PMU	–	Programme Management Unit
PPvCs	–	Peripheral Pharmacovigilance Centres (ASU&H Medicines)
PRAC	–	Pharmacovigilance Risk Assessment Committee
PRISM	–	Post-Licensure Rapid Immunization Safety Monitoring Programm
PSC	–	Project Sanctioning Committee
PSUR	–	Periodic Safety Update Report
PV	–	Pharmacovigilance

PvMF	–	Pharmacovigilance System Master File
PvOI	–	Pharmacovigilance Officer in Charge
PvPI	–	Pharmacovigilance Programme of India
QA	–	Quality Assurance
RCT	–	Randomized Control Trial
RI	–	Routine Immunization
RMP	–	Risk Management Plan
SCTIMST	–	Sree Chitra Tirunal Institute of Medical Sciences and Technology
SDA	–	Signal Detection Algorithm
SPC	–	Siddha Pharmacopoeia Committee
TGA	–	Therapeutic Good Administration
TRRF	–	Transfusion Reaction Reporting Form
UMC	–	Uppsala Monitoring Centre
UN	–	United Nations
UPC	–	Unani Pharmacopoeia Committee
USA	–	United States of America
USD	–	United States Dollar
USFDA	–	United States Food and Drugs Administration
WHA	–	World Health Assembly
WHO	–	World Health Organization
WHO ART	–	WHO Adverse Reaction Terminology
WHO DD	–	WHO Drug Dictionary
YCS	–	Yellow Card System

Chapter 1

Introduction

"The farther back you look the farther forward you can see"

Winston Churchill

After reading this chapter, you should be able to understand and appreciate:
• The genesis and importance of the term 'Pharmacovigilance'.
• The consequences of Adverse Drug Reactions.
• Historical development of safety monitoring programme.
• The sources of data for Pharmacovigilance.
• Aims and Scope of Pharmacovigilance.
• The Minimum Requirements for National Pharmacovigilance System.

Pharmacovigilance is the science of collecting, monitoring, researching, assessing and evaluating information from healthcare providers and patients on the adverse effects of medicines, biological products, herbals and traditional medicines with a view to identify new information about hazards and preventing harm to patients. The word 'Pharmacovigilance' is derived from the Greek word *pharmakon* meaning drug and the Latin word *vigilare* meaning to keep awake or alert, to keep watch. The word was initially used in France in 1960s and later was perceived as the new name for the old terminology post marketing surveillance (PMS). The Pharmacovigilance term is now used internationally. The World Health Organization introduced the term in 2002 and has been adopted by International Conference on Harmonization of Technical Requirements for Registration of Pharmaceuticals for Human Use (ICH).The domain of Pharmacovigilance is not just restricted to PMS but to the entire period of journey of medicines and related products from the pre-approval development to the post approval period.

Safety and efficacy parameters are the prime requirements of evaluation in the process of drug development. While efficacy is important for assessing the usefulness of a testing drug, the safety requirements make it whether to use or not. The possibility that drug use could result in adverse reaction came to the fore rather earlier than did concern about inefficiency. Even, the father of the modern medicine Hippocrates said "Do no harm". There are many quotes which described the importance of safety issues. The two are cited here:

"Cured yesterday of my disease, I died last night of my physician/medicine".

"Go to the Doctor, get your prescription, pay his fees as the doctor has to survive; Go to the Pharmacist, buy your medicine and pay for it, because the pharmacist has to survive; Now go home and throw your medicines because you need to survive".

The quotes are just to emphasize the issues with the use of medicines and they are not to undermine the importance of medicines in everybody's life. The medicines are perhaps the greatest weapon of mankind fighting illnesses, preventing diseases and improving quality of life besides increasing longevity.

The new drugs undergo a significant amount of testing for safety and efficacy in animals and humans through which the effectiveness can be assessed with certainty but the safety issue with less certainty. The clinical trials never tell the whole story of the effects of a drug in all situations. The clinical trials are incomplete studies due to various reasons like limited and selected patients are used; duration of trial is limited; data on special group of patients either not generated or incomplete. The clinical trials can detect only the commonest adverse drug reactions (with more than 1% incidence). The less common adverse drug reactions (with less than 1% incidence) can only be discovered in a long term study in large population. It took decades before the ADRs of Aspirin on gastrointestinal tract became apparent. It also took years to recognise the renal toxicity of phenacetin. This implies the need of continuing drug safety evaluation in post approval period.

The safety study in post approval period is also called post marketing surveillance (PMS). The word surveillance is derived from French terms: *sur* (meaning over) and *veiller* (meaning to watch). The terminology post marketing surveillance first appeared in 1960s and is attributed to Bill

Inman, a medically qualified doctor worked in drug safety issues in UK for long time.

Clinical Trials (CT): *They are human experimentations conducted in order to assess the safety and efficacy of prospective drug. CT is broadly divided into: Pre-approval and post approval studies. Pre-approval studies are divided into Phase – I, Phase – II and Phase – III.*

Phase – I: *is conducted in 20-100 healthy volunteers to determine the tolerable concentration, the route of administration and the initial pharmacokinetic information. It also checks the possible side effects.*

Phase – II: *is conducted in 100-500 patients. It provides information on efficacy, short term tolerability and to determine the dose that best balances between efficacy and safety (tolerability).*

Phase – III: *is conducted in 1000-5000 patients to confirm effectiveness and monitor adverse drug reactions from longer use.*

Based on the three phases of studies, the drug is approved for marketing. The post approval studies, also called Phase – IV or Post Marketing Surveillance, are conducted to identify the undiscovered adverse drug reactions.

With urgent need of novel treatment for diseases like TB, Malaria, and HIV; more and more drug products are expected to be approved on an accelerated and fast track basis. These arrivals are on conditional basis that safety monitoring is to be continued. This situation further necessitate the need of PV system in place to minimise the risk of new treatment.

Consequences of ADRs

Not that all ADRs are very serious but some are definite causes of death, hospitalization, or serious injury. ADRs have two important consequences on the individuals and the health system:

(i) sufferings (including deaths) and prolonged stay at hospital and

(ii) economic impact. ADRs are one of the leading causes of morbidity and mortality.

In USA, 700,000 emergency department visits and 120,000 hospitalizations are due to ADEs annually. USD 3.5 billion is spent on extra medical costs of ADEs annually. At least 40% of costs on ambulatory (non-hospital settings) Adverse Drugs Events management are estimated to be preventable. In UK, some studies showed that the prevalence of hospital admission resulting directly from adverse drug reactions was over 5% and adverse drug reactions accounted for 0.15% of deaths among all admissions. Worldwide on an average 3 to 5% of hospital admissions are attributed to ADRs and 0.32 to 6.7% is the incidence of serious and fatal adverse drug reactions in hospital patients. Due to poor reporting culture much reliable data from India is not available. However, one study from a south Indian hospital [http://www.ncbi.nlm.nih.gov/pubmed/14762985] reported that 3.7% of the hospitalised patients experienced an ADR, 0.7% of the admissions were due to ADRs and 1.8% had a fatal ADR. The average cost of managing an ADR was reported to be Rs. 690/-.

The safety information obtained helps the drug regulating authority to advice on labelling changes to restricting its availability to completely banning the product. Many drugs have been withdrawn from the world market because of actual or perceived safety concern. An estimated one third was withdrawn within two years of launch and a half within five years. Having learnt the importance of safety monitoring of medicines beyond the clinical trials, it may be appropriate to know how the system of safety monitoring has evolved over the years. This is divided into two periods: pre-thalidomide and post thalidomide period.

Pre-Thalidomide Period

The thalidomide disaster changed the world's outlook towards medicines' safety and the world became wiser and started monitoring the medicines in use. This has been a milestone in safety monitoring programme. But there have been records of toxicity caused by the medicines even much before the thalidomide tragedy. Here are few examples of drug safety records that are reported prior to thalidomide: The death of a person during the routine anaesthetic with chloroform in 1848 in north–east England was identified as an episode of ventricular fibrillation. Chloroform was just introduced a year earlier into clinical practice and was known to be better than ether as the former produced less nausea and vomiting. Because of continuing concerns of the public and the profession about the safety of anaesthesia, the Lancet set up a commission which invited doctors in Britain and its colonies to report anaesthesia related deaths. This was viewed as the forerunner of a system of reporting adverse events; the first suspicion that drug might be involved in causing aplastic anaemia was aroused by Labbi and Langlois in 1919 which is around 30 years after the first description of the disease.

In 1934, the role of a drug in the aetiology of agranulocytosis was suggested for the first time.

Though the recording or documenting of toxic effects of medicines has a long history, even in USA there was no assurance of safety and effectiveness of medicines till 1930s. The manufacturers were not in obligation to disclose the contents on the label. The legislation of 1906, Pure Food and Drug Act, was meant just to ensure the purity and consistency of food and drugs and also to ensure the clear and accurate identification of active ingredients. The Act was silent on safety and efficacy. Until 1938, the drugs could still be useless and/or dangerous as long as the label listed the ingredients in a correct manner.

Story of Sulfanilamide Elixir: In 1937, a remedy of sore throat called sulfanilamide elixir manufactured by a small factory in Tennessee was found to be the cause of 107 deaths. As the drug was not soluble in water, it was difficult to form a paediatric preparation. The company, ignorant of toxic aspects of the new solvent, dissolved drug in diethelene glycol. The product had not been adequately tested for safety.

USFDA seized the entire stock before causing further deaths. FDA acted not because the drug was not safe. Safety was not an issue as it was not the requirement (1906 regulation). The FDA acted because the preparation had been mislabelled. Technically an elixir had to contain some quantity of ethyl alcohol and it had none. This was in violation of the law.

But the incident made America to make regulation not only to ensure the safety of the drug but of the whole product.

Following the sulfanilamide elixir issue, there was demand for better legislation for ensuring safety or against the unsafe drugs. In December 1937, US Congress passed the legislation that had been stalled for several years. This new legislation called Federal Food, Drug and Cosmetic (FDC) Act had taken effect in 1938. This Act necessitated the requirement of demonstration that new drugs were safe before they could be marketed commercially.

Post-Thalidomide Period

A direct consequence of thalidomide disaster that occurred in several countries outside USA, the US Government had amended the FDC Act, known as Kefeuver–Harris Amendment of 1960. As a result of this amendment, the drug companies were required to prove that new drugs were effective as well as safe. The safety was not a matter of concern till this time. The physicians were instructed through a federal programme called MedWatch to report to the FDA any instance of adverse effect resulting from use of new drug by their patients.

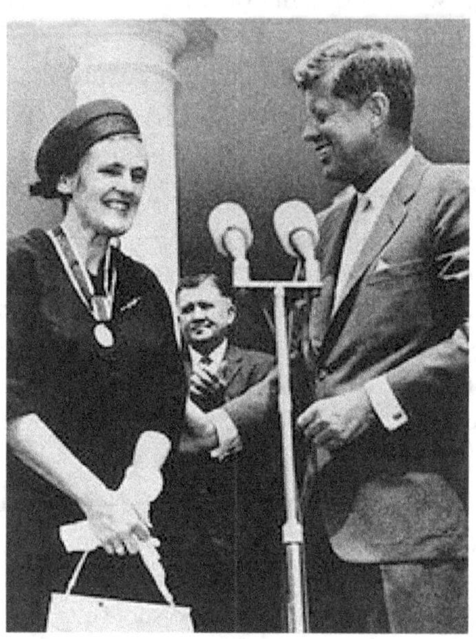

Dr. Frances Kathleen Oldham Kelsey, a pharmacologist in USFDA, prevented the entry of thalidomide into USA market by not approving it. She insisted the need of further studies despite of its approval in UK and other countries. She received commendable appreciation for preventing thalidomide disaster in USA which would have otherwise caused the birth of thousands of armless and legless children. In 1962, she was awarded with President's award for Distinguished Federal Civilian Service from President John F. Kennedy. In 2010 the FDA honoured Kelsey by naming one of their annual awards after her and she was the first recipient.

In UK the Committee on Safety of Drugs (CSD) was formed in 1963. The next year in 1964, it had introduced the Yellow Card system (YCS) with a letter circulated to all doctors urging to report promptly the details of any untoward condition in a patient that might be the result of drug treatment. The YCS is a prepaid system even working today got its name from the colour of the original document used for reporting ADRs. The Medicines and Healthcare Products Regulatory Agency (MHRA) is responsible for ensuring safety and effectiveness of drugs. Committee on Safety of Drugs was replaced by the terminology Committee on Safety of Medicines (CSM) in 1970. Again in 1970, this was replaced by Commission on Human Medicines (CHM).

Again it was felt by World Health Organization (WHO) to have an international system for monitoring adverse reaction to drugs (ADRs) based on the data from national centres. After a pilot study in USA, an international database was established at Geneva, WHO head quarter, in 1971. The base for international monitoring system was moved to Uppsala, Sweden, in 1978. Since then, Uppsala Monitoring Centre (UMC) has been managing the primary aspects of expanding worldwide Pharmacovigilance network of more than 130 countries. UMC is the WHO collaborating Centre for international drug monitoring. India joined the WHO programme in 1998. The Pharmacovigilance Programme of India launched in 2010 has grown leaps and bounds. More than 320,000 reports are contributed to the UMC's VigiBase database (as of 18th September 2018). This is approximately 1.7% of total contribution. The National Coordination Centre, Indian Pharmacopoeia Commission, has achieved the status of WHO Collaborating Centre. The recent initiative of World Health Organization to make the safety database accessible to all would be helpful promoting safe medications.

Minimum Requirements for a Functional National PV System:

1. A National PV Centre with designated at least one full time staff, stable basic funding, clear mandates, well defined structure and roles, and collaborating with WHO Programme for International Drug Monitoring;

2. The existence of a National Spontaneous Reporting System with a National Individual Case Safety Report (ICSR) form;

3. The existence of a National Database or System for collating and managing ADR reports;

4. The existence of National Advisory Committee who should be able to provide technical assistance on causality assessment, risk assessment, risk management, case investigation and where necessary take up management and crisis communication; and

5. The existence of a clear communication strategy for routine and crisis communication.

[Source: The Global Fund to Fight AIDS, TB, and Malaria; and WHO]

Scope of Pharmacovigilance

The scope of PV has expanded and can be diagrammatically presented [WHO Pharmacovigilance Indicators, WHO, 2015]

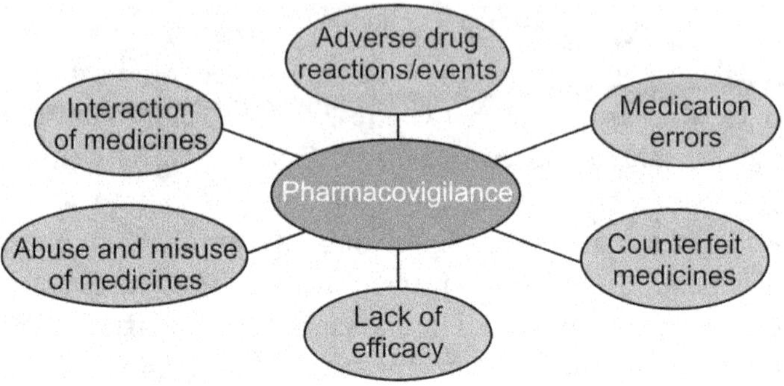

Methods in Pharmacovigilance

The Pharmacovigilance data (ADRs reports) comes primarily from spontaneous reporting (also known as volunteering reporting) by the healthcare professionals. This type of reporting is dependent on the initiative and motivation of the potential reporters, the healthcare professionals. These reports are called "individual case safety report (ICSR)". Another issue with the voluntary reporting that doctors may worry that the adverse effects they report may be seen as the result of their bad practice which may not only leave them open to criticism but also to litigation.

In addition to spontaneous reporting of adverse drug reactions, there are systems/methods to have active surveillance. Usually the academic scientists or hospitals or industries contribute significantly by active follow up after treatment. The events may be detected by asking patients directly or screening patients' records. The cohort event monitoring is the most comprehensive method. The active surveillance is also a part of pharmacoepidemiolgy which is defined as the science of investigating the effects of drugs already in the market in large group of population.

Irrespective of the source of data, the reports are analysed for assessing their association with the drug(s) called causality assessment. They are useful in detecting a signal, a notice of an early concern about possible drug safety problem. Detecting signals is one of the primary objectives of Pharmacovigilance. The Pharmacovigilance data provides evidence for making regulatory decisions based on strengthened signals.

Pharmacovigilance Programme aims to:
- Improve patient care through ensuring safety of medicines;
- Improve public health through ensuring safe use of medicines;
- Help in assessment of benefit, harm, effectiveness and risk of medicines;
- Promote understanding, education, and training on Pharmacovigilance to ensure safe use of medicines [Reducing or minimising medicine use related harm].

Conclusion

Pharmacovigilance aims at getting the best outcome from a drug treatment. Though no one wants to harm patients, unfortunately many medicines harm the patients sometimes. Good Pharmacovigilance will identify the risks in the shortest possible time after the medicine is marketed and will help to establish/identify risk factors. The Pharmacovigilance information would allow intelligent and evidence based prescribing with potential for preventing many adverse reactions. This would ultimately ensure optimum therapy at a lowest cost to each patient and the health system.

Dr. Marie Lindquist, Director of Uppsala Monitoring Centre, compares the Pharmacovigilance activities with observational skills of the Sherlock Homes. With his attention to every detail and its meaning and implication help Sherlock to analyze the situation in logical way and solve the mystery. She quotes Sherlock "when you have eliminated the impossible, whatever remains, however improbable, must be the truth".

Pharmacovigilance Practice requires handling and managing huge volume of data with increasing data complexity. The drug safety industries are looking for solutions to reduce case processing costs without compromising the need of regulatory requirements and quality of information. Artificial Intelligence (AI) and the Cloud Technology offer a solution. The AI will do the work that once only humans could do. The future of PV will depend on automation and machine learning. The system must be geared up before embracing this new change which is inevitable.

While the safety of the medicines and the related products are of prime importance to all stakeholders: manufacturers, health professionals and the patients, falsely attributing a harmful effect to a medicine, or a treatment, causes a lot of damage which can be difficult to reverse. The reported causal relationship between the MMR (Measles, Mumps and Rubella) vaccination and autism influenced the patients rejecting the vaccine. MMR vaccine was introduced in UK in 1988 as a replacement of individual vaccines. Following the study reported in the Lancet in 1998 on the possible link between the autism and MMR vaccine raised an alarm among the parents. This impacted the higher prevalence of measles in the UK. There were 2,016 confirmed cases of measles in England and Wales in 2012, the highest total for 18 years. However, one of the biggest studies of all -a 2002 paper examining the records of 537,303 children born in Denmark - also showed no link between MMR and autism [http://www.bbc.co.uk/news/health-22173393 accessed on 19 October 2013].

Key Messages

- The word 'pharmacovigilance' is originated in France in 1960 from Greek word 'pharmakon' [meaning drug] and Latin word 'vigilare' [meaning to keep watch].

- Though pharmacovigilance originally intended for safety monitoring of approved medicines (post-marketing surveillance), now it includes the safety monitoring for the entire period of life cycle inclusive of pre- approval and post- approval period.

- Pre-approval clinical trials cannot detect all adverse drug reactions but only the common ones with more than 1% incidence. Hence, there is a need of post-marketing surveillance when medicines are used by large section of the population.

- Though all adverse drug reactions are equally harmful affecting human health, they are one of the leading causes of morbidity and mortality worldwide.

- Safety information (Adverse drug reaction reports) collected in pharmacovigilance programme helps the regulatory authority (Government) to take appropriate action ranging from advices on labelling change to restricting availability to completely banning a product.

- Following Thalidomide disaster of 1960s the countries had initiated programme on safety monitoring including the International drug monitoring by WHO. At present 130 countries are participating in WHO's programme.

- India's National Pharmacovigilance Programme is coordinated by Indian Pharmacopoeia Commission.

- Pharmacovigilance aims to ensure safe and optimum therapy.

Bibliography

1. Guru Prasad Mohanta, Textbook on Clinical Research: A Guide for Aspiring Professionals and Professionals, PharmaMed Press, Second Edition, 2017.

2. Management of Safety Information from Clinical Trials, Report of CIOMS Working Group VI, CIOMS, Geneva, 2005.

3. MNG Dukes, Drug Utilization Studies, WHO Regional Publications, 1993.

4. Pharmacovigilance Programme of India Performance Report 2018-2019, Indian Pharmacopoeia Commission, Government of India, 2019.

5. Safety of Medicines, World Health Organization, Geneva, 2002.

6. The Importance of Pharmacovigilance, World Health Organization, 2002.

7. View Point – Part 1, the Uppsala Monitoring Centre, 2002.

8. View Point – Part 2, the Uppsala Monitoring Centre, 2005.

Chapter 2

Pharmacovigilance in India

"The worst thing about medicine is that one kind makes another necessary".

Elbert Hubbard

After reading this chapter, you should be able to understand and appreciate:
• The need and genesis of pharmacovigilance programme in India.
• The salient features of Pharmacovigilance Programme of India [Currently in Operation].
• The functioning of Pharmacovigilance Programme of India.
• Achievements of the Pharmacovigilance Programme of India.
• Regulatory aspects of Pharmacovigilance in India.
• Future Prospects of Pharmacovigilance in India.

The Indian Pharmaceutical Industries have made tremendous progress in terms of infrastructure development, technology base and wide range of products in last few decades. The strength of Indian pharmaceutical industries is in developing cost effective technologies in shortest possible time without compromising qualities. Many of the Indian companies have international regulatory approvals for their plants from agencies like USFDA, MHRA-UK, TGA-Australia, MCC – South Africa etc. The country exports medicines to more than 200 countries including USA, Canada, UK, etc. In fact, the whole world looks for India for cost-effective generic medicines. India is known as Pharmacy of Third World. It is the third largest in the world in terms of volume and 14th in terms of value accounting for around 10% of world's production by volume and 1.5% by value.

India becomes a favourite clinical research destination as there has been increasing focus on cost cutting in drug development process.

Clinical trials seem to be 10-50% cheaper in India compared to the cost involved in developed countries. The booming clinical research in India is evident from India's apex drug regulatory authority's (Central Drug Standard Control Organization) statistics. The number of new Drug Application has increased to 1753 in 2009 from 1200 in 2005. The global clinical trials' number is increased from 100 in 2005 to 262 in 2009 with a peak of 350 in 2008. Safety monitoring of test products during the clinical trials or clinical research is an important requirement. Besides, many new products too are approved for use in India. The safety monitoring of introduced new drugs is mandatory as post marketing surveillance.

The growth of Indian pharmaceutical industries together with rapid growth of clinical research scenario emphasizes the need of a robust safety monitoring programme, Pharmacovigilance Programme. Realising the need of such programme, the Government of India re-launched the massive and ambitious National Pharmacovigilance Programme in 2010 with its own expense. The earlier National Programme was initiated in 2004 with World Bank assistance that stopped functioning in 2008 as the project ended.

> Every country needs to have its own Pharmacovigilance programme not just relies on the International Programme as there are Geographical differences in disease prevalence, Genetic Polymorphism, Healthcare system, Healthcare practices, Indications for use of medicines, Formulation practices and Drug use monitoring practices.

The ADR monitoring programme is not new to India. We could not see much progress till National Pharmacovigilance Programme of India was launched in 2010. In 1982, five centres were established by the Drugs Controller of India. Indian Council for Medical Research (ICMR) had collected about 58,000 reports through its multi-institutional study but they all stopped functioning after few years. In 1989, six regional centres were set up in Bombay, New Delhi, Calcutta, Lucknow, Pondicherry and Chandigarh under the aegis of Drugs Controller of India. In 1987, the India finally joined the WHO ADR monitoring programme with Department of Pharmacology, All India Institute of Medical Sciences (AIIMS) as National Centre and KEM hospital (Bombay) and JLN Hospital, Aligarh Muslim University, Aligarh,as the WHO special centres. These centres and the programme could not be sustained due to lack of adequate funding and other factors.

Though there were lot of enthusiasm in the beginning of World Bank assisted National PV programme, this could not be sustained. There was no full time staff at CDSCO to look after the programme. The outcome or output of the programme was not encouraging. There was lack of communication from top to the bottom in the structure, flow of fund often was the issue and there were other reasons too. This was the first structured programme with prescribed tasks for each centre with monitoring provisions. The merit of the programme was that it had centres from private community pharmacy to pharmacy colleges (with pharmacy practice programme) and medical colleges. The new programme launched later in 2010, at least beginning phase, concentrated only on medical colleges as centres. The details of World Bank assisted National Programme is dropped in the current edition of the text.

Pharmacovigilance Programme of India (PvPI)

Post 2005 there has been tremendous increase in number of applications relating to new chemical entity and their approval by drugs regulatory authority. This is reflected from the CDSCO data: 10,000 applications in 2005 to 22,806 in 2009. The rapid introduction of new drugs and high tech pharmaceutical products to the health care market threw new challenges and this necessitates the need of a nationwide programme to monitor adverse drug reactions. As the World Bank Project ended, the government of India planned to restart the National Pharmacovigilance Programme. With this in mind, a brain storming workshop was organized in the Department of Pharmacology, All India Institute of Medical Sciences (AIIMS) in 2009 in association with CDSCO and WHO Country office for India. This meeting formulated the frame work of the new programme and was operational from mid July 2010. The CDSCO initiated this new PvPI 14 July 2010 with Department of Pharmacology, AIIMS, New Delhi, as the National Co-Ordination Centre. The National Co-Ordination Centre (NCC) has been shifted to Indian Pharmacopoeia Commission, Ghaziabad with effect from 15 April 2011. The NCC operates under the supervision of Steering Committee to recommend procedures and guidelines for regulatory interventions.

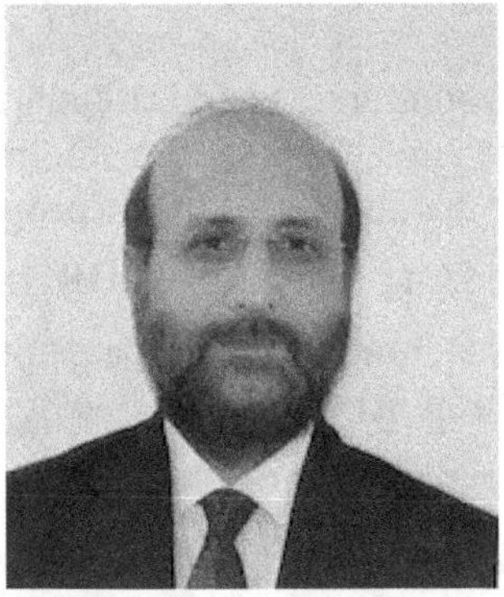

Dr Surinder Singh, Former Drugs Controller General (India), was responsible for re-launching the National Pharmacovigilance Programme in India in 2010 with its own budgetary support. He is also responsible for initiating National Haemovigilance Programme in 2012. Currently Dr. Singh is the Director of National Institute of Biologicals, Government of India (2019).

Supervision

The Steering Committee is consisting of DCGI as *ex-officio* Chairman and Officer in Charge (New Drugs), CDSCO, as *ex-officio* Secretary. In addition it has another 8 members:

1. Scientific Director, Indian Pharmacopoeia Commission, Ghaziabad, *Ex- Officio*,

2. Head, Department of Pharmacology, AIIMS, *Ex- Officio*,

3. Nominee of Director General, Indian Council for Medical Research, *Ex- Officio*,

4. Assistant Director General, Extended Programme of Immunization, as representative of Directorate General of Health Services,

5. Under Secretary (Drugs Control) as representative of the Ministry of Health and Family Welfare,

6. Nominee of Vice Chancellor of Medical / Pharmacy University, *Ex- Officio*,

7. Nominee of Medical Council of India, *Ex- Officio*,

8. Nominee of Pharmacy Council of India, *Ex- Officio*.

Goal and Objectives

The goal of the new programme is to safeguard the health of Indian population through ensuring benefits of medicine use outweighing the risks. The followings are the objectives of the programme:

- To monitor Adverse Drug Reactions (ADRs) in Indian Population.
- To create awareness among healthcare professionals about the importance of ADR reporting in India.
- To monitor benefit-risk profile of medicines.
- To generate independent, evidence based recommendations on safety of medicines.
- To support the CDSCO for formulating safety related regulatory decisions for medicines.
- To communicate finding to all key stakeholders.
- To create a National Centre of Excellence on par with global drug safety monitoring standards.

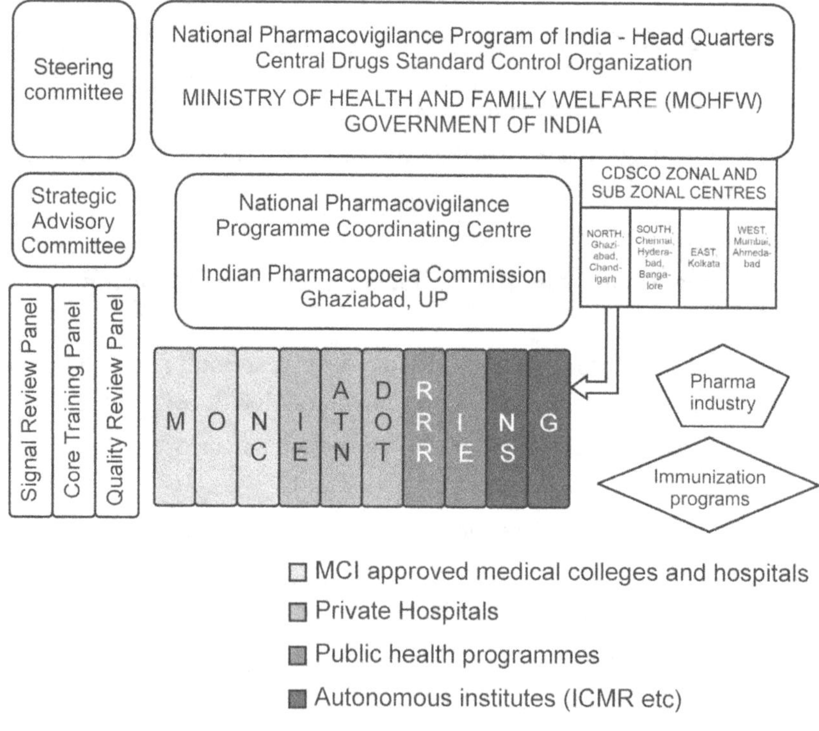

Road Map and Target

The five year road map of the programme (2010 to 2015) had fixed the following targets to achieve:

Period (Phase)	Targets
2010-2011 (Initiation Phase)	Developing systems and procedures. Enrol 40 medical colleges. Start data collection from Adverse Events Following Immunization (AEFI). Development and establishment of training centres. Training of Pharmacovigilance human resource. Linkage with Uppsala Monitoring Centre, Sweden (WHO Collaborating Centre). Initiate software development for National Drug Safety Data Base. Zonal workshops for public awareness of drug safety. Publication of Drug Safety Newsletter.
2011-2012 (Expansion and Consolidation Phase)	Enrol 60 additional medical colleges. Training of Pharmacovigilance human resource. Identify gaps and address through appropriate training. Training on Pharmacovigilance software provided by Uppsala Monitoring Centre (Vigiflow). Software development and validation. Zonal workshops for public awareness of drug safety. Publication of Drug Safety Newsletter.
2012-2013 (Expansion and Maintenance Phase)	Enrol additional 100 medical colleges. Training of Pharmacovigilance human resource. Zonal workshops for public awareness of drug safety. Publication of Drug Safety Newsletter.
2013-2014 (Expansion and Optimization Phase)	Enrol additional 100 medical colleges. Interaction with International Pharmacovigilance Bodies. Training of Pharmacovigilance human resource. Publication of Drug Safety Newsletter.
Excellence Phase (2014-2015)	Create Centre of Excellence for Pharmacovigilance in Asia Pacific.

Operational Principles and Responsibilities of Centres

I. *Centres:* Medical Council of India approved Medical College Hospitals, Private Hospitals, Public Health Programmes and Autonomous Institutes like ICMR are planned to be enrolled as ADR monitoring centres. It is proposed to enrol 300 centres by the end of the five year period.

The medical college centres enrolled under the programme are provided technical, administrative, and financial support by the respective zonal / sub-zonal CDSCO office.

The autonomous institutes/other medical institutes/central institutes are planned to be enrolled on voluntary basis but are not provided any support from CDSCO. Similarly public as well as corporate hospitals are also planned for enrolment on voluntary basis but without any support from CDSCO.

II. *Responsibilities:*

Centre	Functions
Medical College ADR Monitoring Centre	<ul><li>Collection of ADR reports.</li><li>Perform follow up with the complainant to check completeness and as per SOP.</li><li>Data entry into Vigiflow.</li><li>Reporting to National Coordinating Centre through Vigiflow with the source data (original) attached with each ADR case.</li><li>Training / Sensitization / Feedback to physicians through Newsletter circulated by the NCC.</li></ul>
Other Centres (Corporate Hospitals, Autonomous Institutes, Pharmaceutical Industry, Public Health Programmes)	<ul><li>Collection of ADR reports.</li><li>Perform follow up with the complainant to check completeness as per SOP.</li><li>Report the data to CDSCO Head Quarter.</li></ul>
National Coordinating Centre, IPC, Ghaziabad	<ul><li>Preparation of SOPs, guidance documents and training manuals.</li><li>Data collation, Cross check completeness, Causality Assessment etc. as per SOPs.</li><li>Conduct training workshops for all enrolled centres.</li><li>Publication medicines safety Newsletter.</li><li>Reporting to CDSCO HQ.</li><li>Analysis of PMS, PSUR, AEFI data received from CDSCO HQ.</li></ul>
Zonal / Sub-Zonal CDSCO Offices	<ul><li>Provide procurement, financial and administrative support to ADR monitoring centres.</li><li>Report to CDSCO HQ.</li></ul>
CDSCO HQ, New Delhi	<ul><li>Take appropriate regulatory decision and action on the basis of recommendation of NCC (IPC, Ghaziabad).</li></ul>
	<ul><li>Propagation of medicine safety related decisions to stakeholders.</li></ul>

Contd...

	<ul><li>Collaboration with WHO Centre at Uppsala.</li><li>Provide for budgetary provisions and administrative support to run Pharmacovigilance Programme.</li></ul>

III. *Monitoring and Evaluation*:

The programme has identified the various indicators to measure the efficiency of process, outcomes and impact of the programme:

Process indicators

- Number of ADR monitoring centres participating in the programme.
- Number of ADR Monitoring Centre trained in a year.
- Funds budgeted and spent.
- Number of ADR Monitoring Centre Personnel working full time for the programme.

Outcome indicators

- Software platform established.
- Number of ADR reports received in a year.
- Number of ADR reports processed in a year.
- Number of ADR reports submitted to Vigiflow.

Impact indicators

- Number of signals generated and confirmed.
- Number of safety related alerts issued by CDSCO.

The PvPI supports professional staff, designated Technical Associate, to each of the medical college centres with consolidated salary of Rs. 20,000/- per month. The qualification prescribed for Technical Associate are: MBBS / MD in Microbiology / Biochemistry / Pharmacology; or Post Graduate in Biochemistry / Microbiology / Biotechnology / Pharmacy.

As on 31 March 2019 [PvPI Performance Report 2018-2019], the programme has 270 adverse drug monitoring centres. India has the distinction of reporting over one lakh individual case safety reports (ICSRs) to international database and India is currently the 7th largest contributor to the UMC's international drug safety database (Vigibase) with completeness score of 0.94 out of 1 assessed for Indian ICSRs. A copy of the Adverse Drug Reaction Reporting Form is available in Appendix. In order to encourage the reporter, the Indian Pharmacopoeia Commission, the NCC, has introduced the SMS acknowledgement service through a toll free helpline number: 1800 180 3024. The helpline number is available between 9.00 AM to 5.30 PM on Weekdays. The programme is also promoted through social media like Facebook, Twitter, WhatsApp, LinkedIn etc.

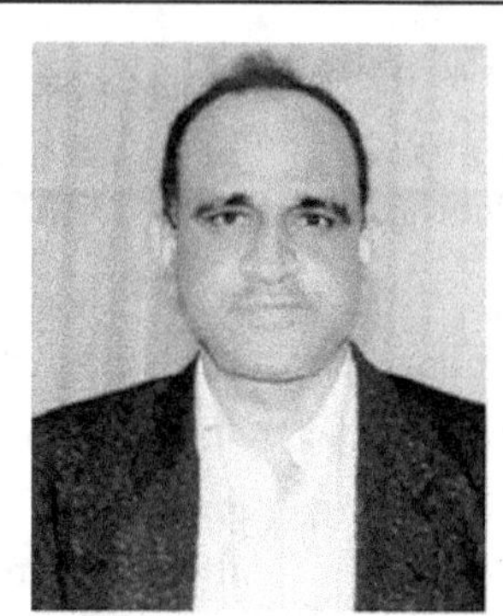

As a Secretary cum Scientific Director, Indian Pharmacopoeia Commission, Government of India, Dr. G. N. Singh was instrumental in strengthening the re-launched National Pharmacovigilance Programme. With his initiative National Coordinating Centre is shifted to the office of Indian Pharmacopoeia Commission, Ghaziabad. Now, he is superannuated (2019).

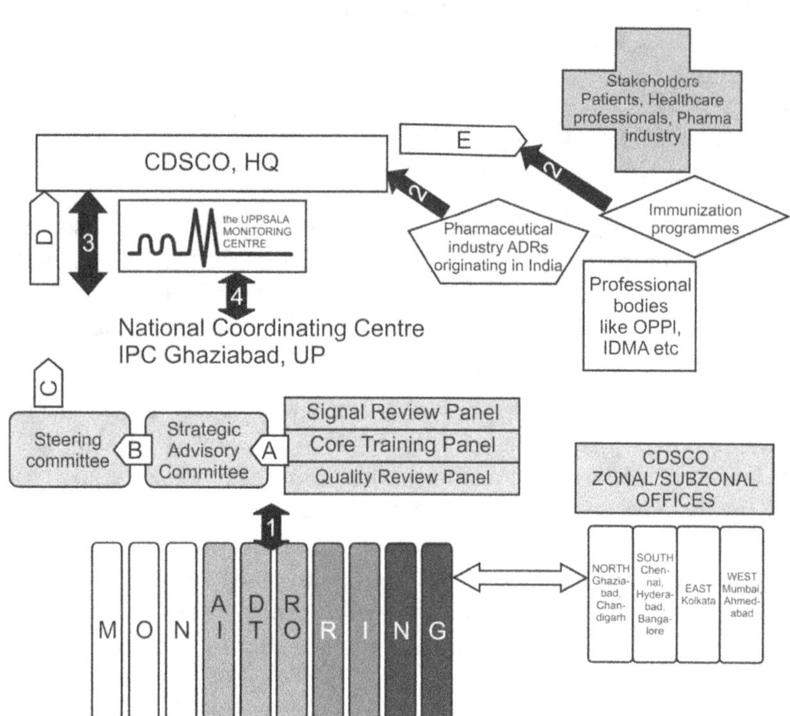

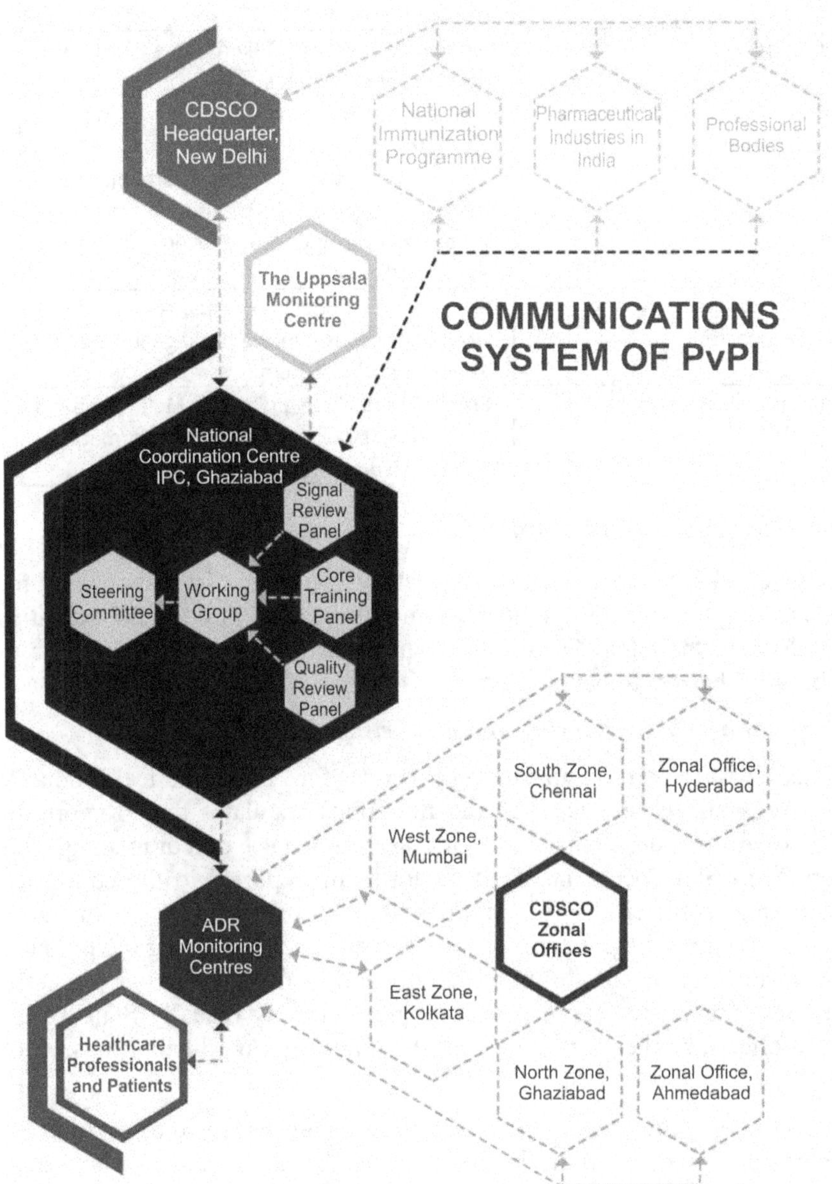

[Source: PvPI Performance Report 2018-2019]

Some Outcomes of PvPI	
Drug (s)	Regulatory Actions Taken based on ADR reports / Label Changes
Carbamazepine Containing Products	Directed to include this in the Prescribing Information: "Initiate screening of HLA-B*1502 prior to initiating the carbamazepine treatment because it is known factor for carbamazepine induced Stevens Johnson's Syndrome".
FDC of Piperacillin and Tazobactam	Directed to include two ADRs: Hypokalaemia and Bronchospasm in the package inserts and other promotional literatures.
Anti-Rabies Vaccine	Directed to include Erythema Multiforme in Drug Safety label in Prescribing Information / Package Inserts.

Regulatory Aspects of PV

CDSCO, the National Drug Regulatory Authority is responsible for conducting the PvPI. Reports and signals generated through PV activities would help the CDSCO to initiate appropriate actions: issuing alerts to labelling changes to banning drugs.

Concerning Manufacturing and Marketing:

Schedule M (Good Manufacturing Practices for Pharmaceutical Products) of Drugs and Cosmetics Act and the Rules stipulates that 'Reports of serious adverse drug reactions resulting from the use of a drug along with comments and documents shall be forthwith reported to the concerned Licensing Authority'. This implies that the marketing authorization holder (pharmaceutical companies responsible for marketing the product) has mandatory responsibility to monitor ADRs related to drugs marketed in the country and report the Licencing Authority (usually State Drugs Controller for other than new drugs) / National Coordination Centre of PvPI.

The company needs to have PV system where the position of Pharmacovigilance Officer in Charge (PvOI) is to be created who would be responsible for PV activities. The qualification specified is either Medical Officer or Pharmacist trained in the collection and analysis of ADR reports. PvOI post is similar to the European Economic Area Qualified Person for PV [EU-QPPV]. The PvOI is responsible for the following tasks:

- Development of training modules and organizing training for staff of PV department;

- Identification of PV activities and framing of SOPs, revision of SOPs;

- Establishment and maintenance of Quality Management System of PV Department [This includes documentation, record control, training and audits]; and

- Responding to queries of Regulatory Authorities [The officer should reside in India].

The MAH needs to report forthwith all serious adverse drug reactions, resulting from the use of drugs, along with comments and documents to the concerned licencing authority.

The Marketing Authorization Holder is responsible for submitting PV System Master File (PvMF). The PvMF must have the following information related to MAH's PV System, details of PvOI, PV Organizational Structure, Sources of Safety Data, PV Processes and PV System's Performance.

Concerning Post Marketing Assessment of New Drug:

The New Drugs and Clinical Trial Rules stipulates that a person intending to import or manufacture any new drug for sale or distribution shall have a PV System in place for collecting, processing and forwarding the adverse drug reaction report to the Central Licensing Authority emerging from use of the drug imported or manufactured or marketed by the applicant in the country. The PV System must have PvOI similar to described earlier. The MAH needs to submit the Periodic Safety Update Report (PSUR) every six months for first two years of approval and for subsequent two years annually. The period may be extended. PSUR, a Risk Management Plan (RMP) and Signal Management results should be submitted at appropriate intervals during the post-marketing phase to monitor the safety and efficacy of the products. More details of PSUR are discussed in a separate chapter.

PV audits and inspections should be conducted both internally and externally to the PV Systems. The audit report is to be documented within the quality system.

Achievements and Challenges: Over the years, there has been tremendous growth of PvPI. Some of the achievements are given below:

- Number of AMC has increased by more than 10 fold from 22 in 2010 to 270 in March, 2019.

- The process of ADR reporting is streamlined and is supported by feedback, circulars, and newsletter.

- More than 320,000 reports are contributed to the UMC's VigiBase database (as of 18th September 2018). This is approximately 1.7% of total contribution.

- The quality of reports is also good as completeness score of reports from India is rated at above 0.8 out of 1 during 2014 to 2015.

- The NCC of PvPI has collaborated with other health programmes: Tuberculosis, AIDS, National Vector Borne Disease, and Deworming Programmes.

- The NCC has collaborated with other medical organizations like ICMR, Indian Medical Association, and National Accreditation Board for Hospitals and Healthcare Providers (NABH) for promoting monitoring and reporting of ADRs.

- Achieved the status of WHO Collaborating Centre: IPC, the NCC, is recognised as First WHO Collaborating Centre for Pharmacovigilance in Public Health Programmes and Regulatory Services. This is the first such collaborating centre of WHO.

Milestones of Development of PV in India			
Year	Description	Year	Description
1983	The first ADR Monitoring Centre was established at Christian Medical College, Vellore, by Dr. Molly Thomas, Clinical Pharmacologist.	2012	Haemovigilance Programme is launched
1986	Formal ADR Monitoring Centres were proposed by the Central Drugs Control Department with 12 Regional Centres.	2015	Materiovigilance Programme is launched.
1989	Six Regional ADR Monitoring Centres were established by DCGI. At the same time ICMR too initiated 12 centres as a multi-centre project to monitor adverse drug reactions.	2016	PV becomes mandatory requirements for Pharmaceutical Industries.

Contd...

1997	India joined WHO's Pharma-covigilance Programme.	2017	National Coordination Centre, Indian Pharmacopoeia Commission, is recognised as WHO Collaborating Centre in Public Health Programmes and Regulatory Services
2004	World Bank supported PV Programme, named as National Pharmacovigilance Programme of India, was launched.	2017	The National Strategic Plan for Scaling up of PV Programme is launched.
2010	Pharmacovigilance Programme of India launched		
2011	Indian Pharmacopeia Commission becomes the National Coordination Centre		

In another new initiative, the National Coordinating Centre, IPC, launched the Android Mobile Application in association with NSCB Medical College, Jabalpur, to further strengthening the National Programme. The application has very interesting in built features which would help the private healthcare professionals to report the adverse events in a simple way.

Several software companies too have ventured into pharmacovigilance and this has increased the skilled manpower requirement for carrying out pharmacovigilance activities ranging from basic case processing to complex functions such as signal detection and analysis. Perhaps India would be favourable destination for global pharmacovigilance activities.

The country has initiated some other programmes: Adverse events monitoring for medical devices called Materiovigilance; Blood Transfusion related adverse events monitoring called Haemovigilance; and Vaccine Pharmacovigilance. They are dealt in separate chapters.

Though PvPI's NCC, has reached to the level of being recognised as WHO Collaborating Centre, still many challenges remain which needs to addressed. Some of them are: Enrolling Community Pharmacies as AMC as self-medication is very common; awareness building among the general public; building centralized PV database; and building momentum for inactive or poorly functioning AMCs.

PvPI sets to expand further. The National Strategic Plan for Scale up PV India aims to establish PV Systems at District Hospitals, Community Health Centres and Primary Health centres under National Health

Mission. The expansion and compliance with regulatory requirements by pharmaceutical industries would create need of large number of PV professionals. The PvPI has already initiated the nationwide skill development programme.

Key Messages

- India is a favourite destination for conducting clinical trials and source of cost effective medicines. It exports medicines to more than 200 countries. With increasing regulatory requirements globally India has the obligation to have its own medicine safety monitoring programme and not just dependent of international programmes. There are geographical differences in Disease prevalence, Genetic polymorphism, Healthcare system, Healthcare practices, Indications for use of medicines, Formulation practices and Drug use monitoring practices. This necessitated the need of National Programme on Pharmacovigilance.

- Central Drugs Standard Control Organisation (CDSCO) is the apex body responsible for safety monitoring programme of medicines.

- Though first initiative of ADR monitoring was made in 1982, the first Nationwide Pharmacovigilance Programme was launched during November 2004 under a capacity building project funded by World Bank. The programme ended in 2008 as the funding stopped. There were lot of concerns too on the outcome of the programme. The programme was structured but failed to make an impact mostly due to poor coordination.

- The National Programme is re-launched as 'Pharmacovigilance Programme of India' in July 2010. Now the programme has budgetary support for sustainability and about 250 ADR Monitoring Centres. During the short period, it achieved the distinction of reporting of more than one lakh individual case safety reports to Uppsala's International Drug Monitoring Database besides good quality of report. Indian Pharmacopoeia Commission is the National Coordination Centre.

- The NCC is recognised as WHO Collaborating Centre for Public Health Programmes and Regulatory Services. NCC has collaboration with National Heath Programmes: TB, HIV, Vector Borne Diseases and Deworming Programmes.

- The amendment of Drugs and Cosmetics Act and the Rules made PV mandatory for all manufacturers and importers. They need to have PV System in place within the company with Pharmacovigilance Officer in Charge.

- PvPI sets to expand to the level of District Hospitals, Community Health centres and Primary health centres under National Health Mission.

- The country has similar programmes for medical devices (materio vigilance), blood and blood products (haemovigilance) and vaccines (AEFI Surveillance).

Bibliography

1. C. Adithan, National Pharmacovigilance Programme, Indian Journal of Pharmacology (editorial), December 2005.

2. Department Related Parliamentary Standing Committee on Health and Family Welfare, 59th Report on the Functioning of the CDSCO, May 2012.

3. http://cdsco.nic.in/html/pharmaco.html accessed on 02 September 2012.

4. http://ipc.nic.in/index1.asp?linkid=222 accessed on 02 September 2012.

5. J. Vijay Venkataraman, Current Status of Pharmacovigilance in India, Pharmabiz, 1st April 2015.

6. Pharmacovigilance Programme of India, Performance Report 2018-2019, Indian Pharmacopeia Commission, 2019.

7. Pipasha Biswas and Arun K Biswas, Setting standards for proactive Pharmacovigilance in India: The way forward, Indian Journal of Pharmacology, June 2007.

8. Safety of Medicines, Pharmacovigilance Programme of India, The Journey travelled and way forward, WHO Drug Information, 32(1), 2018.

9. Urmila M. Thatte, Nayan L. Chaudhari & Nithya J. Gogtay, Pharmacovigilance Program of India: history, evolution and current status, Adverse Drug Reaction Bulletin, No. 312, October 2018.

10. www.cdsco.nic.in accessed on 02 September 2012.

11. Y. K. Gupta, Ensuring Patient Safety – Launching the New Pharmaco-vigilance Programme of India, Pharma Times, August 2010.

Chapter 3

Methods in Pharmacovigilance

"Whatever you do will be insignificant, but it is very important that you do it".

Mahatma Gandhi

After reading this chapter, you should be able to understand and appreciate:
• Concept of active Pharmacovigilance and passive Pharmacovigilance;
• Concept of Various Methods: Spontaneous Reporting, Intensified ADR Reporting, Targeted Reporting, Cohort Event Monitoring, and Electronic Health Record Mining;
• Details of Spontaneous Reporting Method of Adverse Drug Reactions;
• Details of Cohort Event Monitoring Method in Pharmacovigilance; and
• Differences between Spontaneous Reporting and Cohort Event Monitoring.

In simplest way, Pharmacovigilance may be described as the adverse drug events surveillance activity. Based on the surveillance activity the Pharmacovigilance may be divided into: Active Pharmacovigilance and Passive Pharmacovigilance. In Active Pharmacovigilance, active measures are taken to detect the adverse events; and in passive Pharmacovigilance the health professionals and patients are encouraged to volunteer reporting of adverse events.

Active Pharmacovigilance is a prospective surveillance and events are usually detected by active follow up of the patients or their treatment records. It is a systematic approach for more comprehensive data. The Active Pharmacovigilance provides opportunity to obtain denominator of persons exposed to medicines and allowing calculating adverse drug event rates. The methods of Active Pharmacovigilance are: cohort event monitoring, use of registers, record-linkage and screening of laboratory results. Examples of cohort event monitoring: Intensive medicine monitoring programme of New Zealand and prescription event monitoring of England. The Passive Pharmacovigilance relies on spontaneous reporting. The Indian Pharmacovigilance Programme is based on the spontaneous reporting. The spontaneous reporting is the most common method of Pharmacovigilance.

Spontaneous reporting is for the reporting of suspected adverse drug reaction (not events in general) while the cohort event monitoring records all clinical events (not just suspected adverse drug reactions).

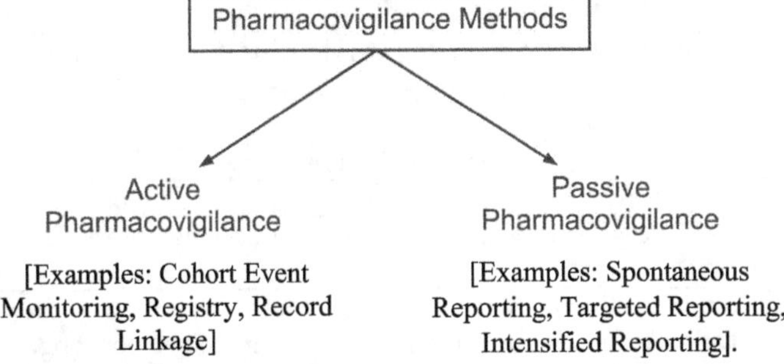

Cohort Event Monitoring (CEM): Cohort event monitoring is a prospective observational cohort study of adverse events associated with one or more medicines. Cohort means a group of people who share a common characteristic like exposure to a drug within a defined time period. The CEM is basically an observational study during routine clinical practice of a new medicine in the early post-marketing phase and aims at detecting early warning(s).

The salient points of CEM are:

- The study is planned prior to beginning of the treatment with the medication(s);

- All patients who receive the particular medication(s) are made part of the study;

- Every patient is followed up for adverse events since the time of treatment;

- All adverse events are to be recorded and not just the suspected adverse reactions: even minor events, change in pre-existing condition, abnormal change in laboratory tests, lack of effectiveness, admission to hospital including deaths etc.;

- It requires two identical groups of patients receiving different treatment; and

- Sample size: The sample size is determined based on expected adverse event incidence. A cohort of 10 thousand patients gives 95% chance   of identifying a specific event with an incidence of 1 in 3000.

The CEM is often inappropriately described as Prescription Event Monitoring [PEM]. The PEM is appropriate when the individual prescription is monitored and the patients receive the medicines based on prescription only. [Patients may also be obtaining medicines without prescriptions].

Example: ADR monitoring of Anti-retroviral medicines. The Government of India launched the ADR monitoring of these medicines under National Pharmacovigilance Programme.

Cohort Event Monitoring	
Pros	**Cons**
Effective in early detection of signals of unsuspected ADRs.	1. Method is more laborious than spontaneous reporting method.
Availability of denominator information allows calculation of incidence rates of ADRs.	2. More expensive method than spontaneous reporting.
Ability to produce a near complete profile of adverse events or adverse drug reactions for the medicines of interest.	3. Being new to health professionals and Pharmacovigilance programme, training is necessary. [Even training is necessary for spontaneous reporting in India as Pharmaco-vigilance is still in its infancy]
Ability to identify and assess risk and risk factors.	4. Long term follow up may be substantial and needs to be actively managed.
Ability to make accurate comparisons between medicines.	
Ability to establish a pregnancy register and identify problems with pregnancy and common congenital abnormalities.	
Ability to record and examine details of all deaths and provide rates of death.	
Being intensive, the method has the ability to provide clinically significant results rapidly.	
With routine follow up, the method has the ability to detect reduced or failed therapeutic effect. It raises the suspicion of inaccurate diagnosis, poor prescribing, inadequate adherence to treatment, emerging resistance or poor quality medicines.	

Registries: A registry is a record of patients with same characteristics. The registries may be disease specific (disease registry), or specific exposure to drug (drug registry) or type of exposure during a specific life event (pregnancy exposure registry). The registry records the information collected prospectively using standardised questionnaires. This is the most common method used to systematically assess post marketing drug issues in pregnancy. The method is also advocated for assessing the safety of anti-malarial medicines.

Record linkage: Record linkage is the method of assembling information contained in two or more records. The medical or pharmacy or any other relevant record is linked to the safety assessment of medicines. The method is useful for studying long term and late complications by linking well documented complication data and equally documented drug use data at individual level. The method involves data collection through searching of different health database using unique patient identifier. In absence of unique identifying number, any other identifying number like hospital number should be used. The availability of computerised pharmacy or medical records has facilitated the record linkage to safety monitoring programme. The following databases are source of information: register of deaths; register of congenital abnormalities; cancer registers; hospital discharge data; medical and pharmacy billing claims etc.

The quality and extent of drug exposure and diagnostic information is important.

Spontaneous reporting system: Spontaneous adverse drug reaction reporting systems are based on suspected adverse drug reactions. The system collects data about suspected ADRs in a central or regional database. Cases are not collected systematically. A spontaneous report is an unsolicited communication by healthcare professionals or consumers that describes one or more ADRs in a patient who was given one or more medicinal products and that does not derive from a study or any organized data collection scheme. The emphasis is on new findings. The India's National programme does not restrict to only new findings but encourages reporting any reactions that are suspected to be ADR. This helps promoting reporting culture. The terminology 'spontaneous report' is being replaced by individual case safety report.

While different countries or different programmes use different reporting forms, there is need of minimum information for a report to be acceptable. The basic information should be:

- An identifiable source of information / reporter: Name, contact details and status – physician, pharmacist, nurse or patient.

- An identifiable patient: Full name for accurate identification for follow up and to avoid duplication. An identifiable number (if available) and other details like gender, age, weight and height are useful.

- Name(s) of suspected product(s): Brand and Generic Names with dosage form is essential. The dose, mode of administration and indications for use are useful. All other medicines taken at the time of event should also be recorded.

- A description of suspected reaction(s): Date of onset along with a brief clinical description of reaction is essential. Laboratory results (if available), outcome of events (resolved, resolving, no change, death with date etc.) and effect of re-challenge, if any, are useful.

The spontaneous reporting is the most common adverse drug reaction monitoring system and in many countries like India, it is voluntary. Though main limitation of spontaneous reporting systems is their inability to quantify the risk due to non-availability of denominator value, they are the important form of evidence for drug withdrawal or regulatory decisions. Note that all ADRs are not reported; only few are reported.

Examples: Lactic acidosis associated with the biguanides (metformin) was identified.

The form used by National Pharmacovigilance Programme is included in the appendix.

Intensified ADR reporting: This is an extension of spontaneous reporting programme and aims to enhance ADR reporting of specific medicines in early post marketing phase. The procedure is usually followed for new drugs, biological medicines, conditionally approved medicines under exceptional cases, medicines that require additional studies (rare side effects observed during clinical trials). Example: Pharmacovigilance of Antiretroviral medicines under a separate programme.

Targeted spontaneous reporting: This is followed to know more about ADR profile of a specific medicine in the population or to estimate the incidences of a known ADR for a specific medicine in a population. Example: Monitoring renal toxicities related to use of tenofovir based regimen in antiretroviral therapy.

Reasons for inadequate rate of ADR reporting: Dr. Bill Inman described the reasons as seven deadly sins:

1. The mistaken believe that only safe drugs are approved for use.
2. Fear of litigation.
3. A sense of guilt for having caused harm.
4. Ambition to collect and publish a personal series of cases.
5. Ignorance of mechanism for reporting suspected reaction.
6. Diffidence about reporting a mere suspicious.
7. Lethargy or indifference to doctor's responsibility to contribute to the general advancement of knowledge.

Spontaneous Reporting	
Pros	**Cons**
1. Covers the whole population	1. Inherent under reporting – Even in developed countries less than 5% reactions are reported.
2. Includes all medicines	2. Captures only suspected ADRs
3. Continual monitoring through-out the life cycle of a medicine	3. Reporting bias – Seriousness, Severity, Publicity of specific ADRs
4. Details signals of new, rare and serious ADRs can be obtained	4. Difficult to detect – Delayed ADRs
5. Most commonly used Pharma-covigilance method	5. Difficult to calculate reliable rate and measure risk factors
6. Easiest method to establish	6. Deaths are poorly reported
7. Relatively inexpensive compared to CEM	7. Special studies necessary to get accurate information on areas of particular interest – Pregnancy, Paediatrics. The special studies require more funds and thus reduce the cost advantage of spontaneous reporting.
8. Least labour intensive	

Electronic Health Record [EHR] Mining: The electronic health or medical records are rich source of ADR data. They contain detailed patient information and copious longitudinal data. The EHR has emerged as new source that can provide important information which can either complement or improve ADR monitoring programme. The EHR data usually consists of information associated with the process of care and not focusing on adverse drug events. Therefore, ADEs are often sparse in EHR data compared to other types of clinical information: treatments, disorders and symptoms. Besides, the use of EHR for Pharmacovigilance is a new research approach. The signals generated through EHR based different data mining algorithms require further validation. The detailed discussion is beyond the scope of this introductory text.

The comparative characteristics/usefulness of various methods used in Pharmacovigilance are given in the table:

Method	Medicine	Population	Report
Spontaneous Reporting	All medicines – during entire life cycle	All exposed individuals but denominator not known	All suspected ADRs
Intensified Reporting	Specific medicines	All exposed individuals but denominator not known	All suspected ADRs
Targeted Reporting	Specific medicines	Defined Cohort	All suspected ADRs including specific ADRs
CEM	Specific medicines	Defined Cohort	All events
EHR Mining	All medicines	Defined Cohort	All events

Key Messages

- Active Pharmacovigilance refers to the active measures taken to detect adverse events. Passive Pharmacovigilance refers to spontaneous or voluntary reporting of adverse events.

- Spontaneous reporting is for the reporting of suspected adverse drug reaction (not events in general) while the cohort event monitoring records all clinical events (not just suspected adverse drug reactions).

- Cohort event monitoring, an active Pharmacovigilance programme, compares the incidence of particular adverse event in two identical groups one group taking the medicine of interest while the other group is taking different medicine. It indicates the relative risks.

- All medicines are subject to spontaneous reporting while selected medicines that are to be used widely and are of public health importance are subjected to CEM wherever possible.

- Denominator (number of persons exposed to drug) useful in calculating the risk rate is not known in spontaneous reporting but is known in CEM.

- Spontaneous reporting is the most commonly used method in Pharmacovigilance and India's National Programme follows this method.

Bibliography

1. A Practical Handbook on the Pharmacovigilance of Antiretroviral Medicines, World Health Organization, 2009.

2. Good Pharmacovigilance Practice Guide, Medicines and Healthcare Products Regulatory Agency, Pharmaceutical Press, 2010.

3. J. Krska and AR Cox, Adverse drug reactions in Clinical Pharmacy and Therapeutics (Edt by Roger Walker and Cate Whittlesea), Fifth Edition, Churchil Livingstone, Elsevier, 2012.

4. Patrick Waller, An introduction to Pharmacovigilance, Wiley –Blackwell, 2010.

5. Tanzania Food and Drugs Authority's Pharmacovigilance Training Manual for Healthcare Professionals, Second Edition, 2011.

Chapter 4

Adverse Drug Reactions: Classification, Mechanisms and Susceptibility

"Cured yesterday of my disease, I died last night of my physician/medicine"

After reading this chapter, you should be able to understand and appreciate:
• The types of reactions and their attributes.
• The mechanism of such reactions.
• Predisposing factors responsible of ADRs.

The main aim of the Pharmacovigilance programme is to identify the unknown adverse reactions of the medicines. The identification of the ADRs is facilitated by understanding their attributes and the classification. The understanding of classification systems help all stake holders of safety monitoring programme developing strategies on avoidance and management of ADRs.

Classification: The Adverse Drug Reactions can be classified in several ways.

Rawlins-Thompson classification: The simplest way of classifying is to divide them into categories: Type A and Type B based on pharmacology: Dose related or non-dose related reactions. This is also called Rawlins-Thompson classification. The type A reactions are related to the known pharmacology of the drug and are dose related. They are reversible on withdrawal of the drug or even simply after dose reduction. The type A reactions are very common accounting about 80% of the total ADRs. In contrast, the type B reactions are qualitatively different from the normal pharmacological action. They are bizarre and cannot be predicted. They cannot be reproduced in animal models too. Thereafter the basic classification is further divided making ADRs into six types: that means four different types – C, D, E and F are added to the system. Type C is dose related and time related, type D is time related and delayed, type E is related to withdrawal reaction and type F is related to unexpected failure of therapy. Type C reactions usually appear during chronic therapy and show a picture less typical for a drug reaction but mimic natural disease. The type D reactions appear long after a treatment or even skipping a generation. Type E reactions can occur after stopping treatment. Type F reactions means failure of efficacy and such reactions are common. The characteristics of each type with examples and management methods are given in the following table.

Type of Adverse Drug Reaction	Attributes	Examples	Management
Type A [Dose Related] / also known as Augmented	• Common [High incidence] • Related to Pharmacological action [Dose dependent] • Predictable • High Morbidity • Low Mortality • Variable severity but usually mild • Reversible	• Bleeding with warfarin • Hypoglycaemia with sulphonyl-ureas • Headache with glyceryltrinitrate • Bradycardia associated with beta-adrenergic receptor antagonist • Bronchospasm with betablocker use	• Reduction of dose or withholding the drug
Type B [Non-Dose Related] / Also known as Bizarre	• Uncommon [Less incidence] • Unrelated to Pharmacological action [Not dependable on dose] • Unpredictable • Low Morbidity • Variable severity but proportionately more severe than Type A • Irreversible	• Anaphylaxis with penicillin • Hepatitis with halothane • Agranulocytosis with clozapine • Aplastic anaemia caused by chloramphenicol	• Withholding and avoiding in future

Contd...

Type of Adverse Drug Reaction	Attributes	Examples	Management
Type C [Dose Related and Time Related] / Chronic	• Uncommon [Less incidence] • Related to Cumulative dose	• Adrenal suppression with corticosteroids • Osteoporosis with oral steroids	• Reducing the dose or withholding the drug
Type D [Time Related] /Delayed	• Uncommon [Less incidence] • Usually dose related • Appears sometime after use of drug	• Tardive dyskinesia with neuroleptics • Carcinogenesis: DES causing vaginal cancer to next generation members.	Often intractable
Type E [Withdrawal Symptoms]	• Uncommon [Less incidence] • Appears soon after the withdrawal of the drug	• Withdrawal reactions with benzodiazepines • Opiate withdrawal syndrome • Myocardial ischemia after beta-blocker withdrawal	Reintroduction and slow withdrawal of the drug
Type F [Unexpected Failure of Therapy]	• Common (High incidence] • Dose related • Often caused by drug interactions	• Failure of oral contraceptive in presence of enzyme inducer • Resistance to antimicrobials	• Increasing dosage • Provision of concomitant therapy

The above classification is based on the properties of the drug (known pharmacology) and the dose dependence of its effects. It does not take into account some other important factors like: properties of the reactions (the time course of its appearance and severity) and factors accounting for individual variation (genetics, pathological).

> **A drug may cause both type A and type B adverse drug reactions.** Examples - Chlorpromazine [Sedation (A), Cholestatic Jaundice (B)]; Phenytoin [Ataxia (A), Hepatitis (B)] and Warfarin [Bleeding (A), Breast Necrosis (B)]

Though traditionally it is believed that the immunological effects are not dose related but here are some examples that clearly established the dose – response relationship: Hay fever in response to high pollen counts, desensitization by use of increasing dose of cephalosporin. It is, therefore, inappropriate to comment that the type B reactions are not dose dependent.

DoTS system: This three dimensional system was proposed in 2003 by Aroson and Ferner. As the name suggests, the classification is based on three parameters: dose relatedness, time course and susceptibility. The DoTS system classification provides useful means to examine the various factors that describe a reaction and the individual patient's susceptibility.

Dose relatedness: Many adverse drug reactions are related to dose of the drug. In DoTS, the adverse drug reactions are divided into three categories based on dose: toxic effects due to supra-therapeutic dose; collateral effects at standard therapeutic dose; and hyper-susceptibility reactions occurring at sub-therapeutic doses.

Examples: Increased risk of digitalis toxicity with increasing dose [toxic effects]; Osteoporosis due to Corticosteroids [collateral effects]; and Anaphylaxis due to penicillin [hyper-susceptibility reactions].

Time relatedness: The appearance of pharmacological action (including adverse drug reaction) is dependent on concentration of the drug at the site of action and the time at which the drug reaches the site of action.

Examples: Furosemide induces greater diuresis while given as infusion compared to administration as bolus even the dose is same. The toxicity of methotrexate is greater when a low dose is given repeatedly compared to the same amount given as one dose. The reactions can be classified further into time independent reactions and time dependent reactions.

Time independent reactions occur at any time within the treatment period irrespective of duration of treatment. Example: Digoxin toxicity when renal function worsens [Due to change in drug concentration]; and Digoxin toxicity in association with potassium depletion [Action changed without change in concentration].

Time dependent reactions range from rapid and intermediate reactions to delayed reactions. But these terminologies: rapid, immediate and delayed are not clearly defined.

Examples: Rapid reactions [Red man syndrome with vancomycin]; intermediate reactions [Thrombocytopenia due to quinine]; and delayed reactions [Vaginal adenocarcinoma in women who were exposed to diethylstilbestrol in uterus].

Susceptibility: Some persons are more susceptible to adverse reactions than others. The following factors responsible for this susceptibility includes: genetic predisposition, age, gender, altered physiology, disease and drug interaction.

The DoTS system of classification is given in the following table:

Dose relatedness	Time relatedness	Susceptibility
• Toxic effects • Collateral effects • Hyper-susceptibility reactions	• Time independent • Time dependent: • Rapid reactions • Early reactions • Intermediate reactions • Late reactions • Delayed reactions	• Contributing Factors: • Genetic variation • Age • Gender • Altered physiology • Drug interaction • Disease
Example: Anaphylaxis due to penicillin 　• Dose – Hyper-susceptibility 　• Time – First dose 　• Susceptibility – Requires previous sensitization		
Example: Osteoporosis due to corticosteroids 　• Dose – Collateral effect 　• Time – Late 　• Susceptibility – Age and Gender		
Example: Hepatotoxicity due to Isoniazid 　• Dose – Collateral effect 　• Time – Intermediate 　• Susceptibility – Genetic (drug metabolism), age, alcohol, disease		

The DoTS approach has more acceptability as it redresses the issue of some ADRs not fitting into A to F scheme.

It may be appreciated that it may not be possible to classify an ADR into one of the categories discussed above; there may be possibility of expanding or revising the classification further to accommodate the new ADR as identified.

The Adverse Drug Reactions can also be classified on following basis:

The reactions that may occur in any one:

- Drug overdose: Toxic effects associated with over dosing or due to less elimination. Paracetamol hepato-toxicity at high dose (exceeding 4 g daily)

- Drug side effect: Undesirable pharmacologic effects at recommended dose. Anti-histamins cause sedation.

- Drug interaction: Effect of one drug on the effectiveness or toxicity of the other drug. Ferrous sulphate reduces the absorption of tetracycline causing reduced effectiveness of the latter.

Contd...

The reactions that may occur in susceptible individuals:

- Drug intolerance: A low threshold to the normal pharmacological action of a drug.
- Drug idiosyncrasy: A genetically determined, qualitatively abnormal reaction to a drug related to a metabolic or enzyme deficiency.
- Drug allergy: An immunologically mediated reaction, characterised by specificity, transferability by antibodies or lymphocytes, and recurrence on re-exposure.
- Pseudo allergic reaction: A reaction similar to allergic reaction but differs in specificity.

The ADRs at what frequency they affect the people (based on incidence):

- Very Common (incidences in more than 10% exposure),
- Common (incidences in 1% to 10% exposure),
- Uncommon (incidences in 0.1% to 1% exposure),
- Rare (incidences in 0.01% to 0.1% exposure) and
- Very Rare (incidences at less than 0.01% exposure).

Mechanisms of adverse drug reactions: The knowledge of mechanisms of adverse drug reactions helps in avoiding ADRs during medicine use. While it is difficult to categorise the mechanisms into discrete categories, they may be grouped into the following main types:

1. Pharmacological (Physiological) effects.
2. Drug – Drug Interactions.
3. Triggering an immunological action.

The genetic variation and pathological conditions too influence the occurrence of ADRs.

Pharmacological (Physiological) effects: Examples – Non-steroidal anti-inflammatory drugs or corticosteroids may cause gastric haemorrhage or peptic ulcer. Aspirin, an anti-inflammatory agent, may cause bleeding due to its anti-platelet effect. Barbiturates are sedatives but can cause respiratory depression. Antihistamins have sedation as adverse effects.

The drug may cause its effects at another site (which is not desired). Glyceryl trinitrate (used in angina) may cause headache.

The individual's ability to process the drug (including the formulation design) and the pharmacokinetic parameters are also responsible for ADRs. A change in drug formulation may affect the bioavailability. A change in formulation in phenytoin capsule (calcium sulphate is replaced by lactose as diluent) was responsible for causing neurological disorders in 1960s due to increased phenytoin concentration in blood. Impairment in drug metabolism or drug elimination may lead to accumulation of drug in the body causing toxicity.

Drug – Drug interactions: Patients on polypharmacy are more likely to have ADRs. All the three types of drug interactions – pharmaceutical, pharmacodynamic and pharmacokinetic interaction may cause ADRs (may increase toxicity or reduce therapeutic efficacy). An Angiotensin Converting Enzyme (ACE) inhibitor and a potassium sparing diuretic, if given together, may result in hyperkalaemia and cardiac arrhythmias. Cimetidine inhibits the metabolism of warfarin and thereby increases the latter's anti-coagulant effect leading to bleeding.

Triggering an immunological action: This leads to allergic or hypersensitivity reactions. These types of reactions do not resemble pharmacological actions. Drug either alone or in combination with antigenic proteins precipitates allergic reactions. The severity of allergic reaction, in general, related to the route of administration. Anaphylactic shocks are more common with injections. Injection of penicillin may cause anaphylaxis. Hence, penicillin allergy is always tested before giving the full dose. Many drugs cause skin allergy like pruritus. Some may cause fatal Stevens – Johnson Syndrome.

Susceptibility to adverse drug reactions: Some people are more susceptible than others to ADRs due to presence of risk factors. The knowledge of the risk factors provides an opportunity for avoiding or minimizing the number of adverse effects and also reducing the harm to the patients. The risk factors that are responsible for susceptibility to ADRs can be grouped into three categories: factors associated with the patient; factors associated with the medicine; and factors associated with the environment.

Risk factors associated with the patient

- **Age:** The elderly and neonates are at greatest risk. The elderly persons, with age related decline in metabolism and elimination coupled with co-morbid conditions, are more susceptible to ADRs. A decreased volume of distribution and decreased rate of elimination result in increased drug concentration which in turn increases the probability of adverse drug effects.

  Example: All central nervous system depressants are liable to have greater effect than normal leading to confusion. Barbiturates may lead to immobility. Flucloxacillin induced jaundice and hepatitis is more common in elderly persons.

Children differ from adults in terms of body composition; and the ability to metabolize and eliminate. The immature blood – brain barrier makes the children more sensitive to morphine. Example – Aspirin is associated with Reye's syndrome in children.

- *Size, weight and height or body mass index:* The normal doses are designed based on average adult body weight of 70 kg. Such dose may result in higher drug concentration in those of lower body weight leading to drug toxicity.

- *Genetic polymorphism:* Patients' genetic makeup makes them more susceptible to ADRs.

  Example: Stevens-Johnson Syndrome and Toxic Epidermal Necrolysis are associated with carbamazepine and phenytoin and more common in population of China, Thailand, Malaysia, Indonesia, the Philippines and Taiwan than people of India and Japan. The readers are advised to read the chapter on Pharmacogenetics.

- *Gender (pregnancy):* Women are generally at higher risk.

  Examples: Thalidomide's association with birth defects. The psychiatric adverse events with mefloquine are more common in females.

- *Co-morbidities:* The co-morbidities such as congestive cardiac failure, respiratory disorders, diabetes, hepatic, renal impairment etc., have profound influence on drug action. The respiration depressant drugs [opiates, barbiturates] may precipitate respiratory failure in patients with a malfunctioning respiratory centre [raised intracranial pressure]. The patients with raised intracranial pressure may be restless. The respiratory depressant, if used for quietening the restlessness, may cause respiratory failure.

  Digitalis causes cardiac arrhythmia in patients with myocardial infarction.

- *Renal or Liver damage:* Reduction in hepatic and renal function substantially increases the risk of ADRs.

Risk factors associated with medicine

- *Dose:* Higher the dose more is the risk. Paracetamol exceeding daily dose of 4 g increases the risk of liver toxicity.

- *Duration of therapy:* Benzodiazepine dependence occurs when treatment last several months or years. When the drug is suddenly stopped withdrawal symptoms appear.

- ***Previous exposure:*** Hypersensitivity to penicillin occurs due to prior exposure.

- ***Polypharmacy:*** The use of multiple medicines simultaneously increases the chances of potential interaction.

Risk associated with environment

- ***Tobacco use:*** Smoking increases the enzyme activity in the liver. Smoking increases the removal of theophyline requiring dose adjustment. Smoking decreases the absorption of insulin leading to delayed action. Smokers do require higher dose of glibenclamide.

- ***Alcohol or other drugs:*** Alcohol increases the risk of liver toxicity of paracetamol. There is increased risk of gastric irritation and bleeding with aspirin when taken together with alcohol.

- ***Diet:*** Grape fruit juice is an enzyme inhibitor. When taken with calcium channel blocker, the grape fruit increases the plasma concentration leading to adverse effects.

- ***Medicines of other system:*** A herbal medicine, St. John's Wort, is an enzyme inducer and reduces the effectiveness of ciclosporin.

Key Messages

- The ADRs can be classified at least in two basic ways:
  - Rawlins – Thompson Method: Type A, B, C, D, E and F. Type A is related to pharmacologic action and is dose dependent. Type B not related to pharmacology of the drug and is dose independent.
  - DoTS System: Dose relatedness, Time relatedness and Susceptibility.
- The mechanisms for ADRs: Pharmacological effects, Drug-Drug interactions and Triggering an immunologic action.
- The risks factors that make a person more vulnerable to ADRs are:
  - Patient related factors – age, weight, body mass index, genetic polymorphism, gender, co-morbidities, renal and liver damage;
  - Medicine related factors – dose, duration, previous exposure, and polypharmacy;
  - Environment related factors – tobacco use, alcohol intake, diet and medicine of other system.

Bibliography

1. J K Aronson and R E Ferner, Joining the DoTS: new approach to classifying adverse drug reactions, British Medical Journal, Nov 22, 2003.

2. Patrick Waller, An Introduction to Pharmacovigilance, Wiley – Blackwell, UK, 2010.

3. Roger Walker and Cate Whittlesea (Editors), Clinical Pharmacy and Therapeutics, 5th Edition, Churchil Livingston, Elsevier, 2012.

4. Ronald D. Mann and Elizabeth Andrews (Ed), Pharmacovigilance, Second Edition, John Wiley & Sons Limited, England, 2007.

Chapter 5

Assessment of Adverse Events' Reports

"I firmly believe that if the whole of the material medica, as now used, could be sunk to the bottom of the sea, it would be all better for mankind and the all the worse for the fishes".

Oliver Wendell Holmes

After reading this chapter, you should be able to understand and appreciate:
• Methods of severity assessment of suspected ADR.
• Methods of causality assessment of suspected ADR.
• Methods of preventability assessment of suspected ADR and strategies available to prevent ADRs in health facilities.

The functions of any Pharmacovigilance programme includes monitoring, detecting, reporting, evaluating, and documenting medicine safety data and providing feedback to the reporters, health professionals and the drug regulators. Once the information is collected they need to be analysed to determine the adverse events severity, probable causality and preventability.

Severity: The severity of adverse drug reaction may be classified as:

- *Severe*: Example – Reaction is fatal or life threatening;
- *Moderate*: Example – Reaction requires antidote, medical procedure, or hospitalization;
- *Mild*: Example – the symptoms require only the discontinuation of the drug therapy; and
- *Incidental*: Example – There are very mild symptoms where the patients can choose whether to continue medicine or discontinue.

The severity assessment is best done using modified Hartwig and Siegel scale. The details are given in the tabular form:

Category	Level	Characteristics
Mild	Level - 1	• The ADR requires no change in the treatment with the suspected drug. OR
	Level - 2	• The ADR requires that the suspected drug be withheld, discontinued, or otherwise changed. • No antidote or other treatment is required. • There is no increase in length of hospital stay.
Moderate	Level – 3	• The ADR requires that the suspected drug be withheld, discontinued, or otherwise changed. • An antidote or other treatment is required. • There is no increase in length of stay, OR
	Level – 4	• (a) Any level-3 ADR that increases the length of stay at least by one day. OR
		• (b) The ADR is the cause of admission.
Severe	Level - 5	• Any level- 4 ADR that requires intensive medical care. OR
	Level – 6	• The ADR causes permanent harm to the patient. OR
	Level - 7	• The ADR either directly or indirectly leads to the death of the patient.

Causality: After identifying a suspected ADR, it is important to demonstrate a causal relationship between the drug and the untoward clinical event. Establishing causality is a process which begins by examining the relationship between the drug and the event. Causality assessment is used to determine the likelihood that a drug caused a suspected ADR. There are a number of methods used to judge causation with each one having its own merits and demerits. The methods require some level of expert judgement to apply.

'World Health Organisation' and the 'Naranjo Probability' Scale are simple to apply. They are generally accepted and most widely used methods for causality assessment in clinical practice. These two methods offer objective, reliable and valid causality assessment of ADRs along with the convenience of being easy to apply methods.

WHO causality categories: There are six standardised causality categories designed by WHO: certain (or definite), probable, possible, unlikely, unclassified (or conditional), and un-assessable (or unclassifiable). With the permission of World Health Organization, the characteristics requirements for each causality category are reproduced from *A Practical Handbook on the Pharmacovigilance of Antiretroviral Medicines, 2009*:

Category	Requirements for inclusion in a specific category
Certain (or, definite)	1. The event is a specific clinical or laboratory phenomenon. 2. The time elapsed between the administration of the drug and the occurrence of the event is plausible. [Requirements: dates of drug administration and the date of onset of the event must be known] 3. The event cannot be explained by concomitant disease or any other drug or chemical. [Requirement: Details of other medicines taken must be known. The report must also state if there were no other medicines in use. If this is unknown, then doubt exists and the event cannot be included in this category). 4. The patient recovered within a plausible length of time following withdrawal of the drug. [The date of withdrawal of the drug and the time taken for recovery should be known. If these dates are unknown, then doubt exists and the event cannot be included in this category.] 5. The same event recurred following re-challenge with the same drug alone. [Requirement: The report must state the outcome of re-challenge. If this is unknown, then doubt exists and the event cannot be included in this category.] *It cannot be classified as Certain if there has been no re-challenge, or the outcome of the re-challenge is unknown.*
Probable	1. The event is a specific clinical or laboratory phenomenon. 2. The time elapsed between the administration of the drug and the occurrence of the event is plausible. [The dates of drug administration and the date of onset of the event must be known.] 3. The event cannot be explained by concurrent disease or any other drug or chemical. [The details of other medicines taken must be known. The report must also state if there were no other medicines in use. If this is unknown, then doubt exists and the event cannot be included in this category.] 4. The patient recovered within a plausible length of time following withdrawal of the drug. [The date of drug withdrawal and the time taken for recovery should be known.] 5. Re-challenge did not occur, or the result is unknown. *It cannot be classified as Probable if there has been no de-challenge or the result of de-challenge is not known or the outcome of the event is unknown or if there are other possible causes of the event.*

Contd...

Category	Requirements for inclusion in a specific category

Possible	1. The time elapsed between the administration of the drug and the occurrence of the event is plausible. [The date of administration and the date of onset of the event must be known.]
	2. The outcome of withdrawal of the suspect medicine is not known, and/or medicine might have been continued and the final outcome is not known; and/or
	3. There might be no information on withdrawal of medicine; and /or
	4. The event could be explained by concomitant disease or use of other drugs or chemicals; and / or
	5. There might be no information on the presence or absence of other medicines.
	6. Deaths cannot be coded as probable because there is no opportunity to see the effect of the withdrawal of the drug. If there is a plausible time relationship, a death should be coded as possible.
	7. In addition to deaths, there is a further group of events that do not fit the relationship assessment process and the coding can vary. Consider the following examples:
	  • Myocardial infarction: Many patients recover from this event as part of the natural history of the disease and with very few exceptions, recovery is not a response to withdrawal of a drug. Hence the result of 'de-challenge' is meaningless. This type of reaction may be coded as 'possible'.
	  • Stroke: Some patients recover fully, some partially, some remain severely disabled and some die. All these outcomes are part of the natural history of the disease and, with very few exceptions, are unrelated to drug withdrawal. Again, the result of 'de-challenge' is usually meaningless. This type of reaction may be coded as 'Possible'.
	  • Acute anaphylaxis immediately following an injection: Here there is an obvious direct relationship, but the usual parameters for establishing relationship, e.g., de-challenge do not apply. In this example, best category for relationship is 'certain'.

Unlikely	1. The event occurred with a duration to onset that makes a causal effect improbable with the drug being considered. [The pharmacology of the drug and the nature of the event should be considered in arriving at this conclusion]; and /or

Contd...

Category	Requirements for inclusion in a specific category
	2. The event commenced before the first administration of the drug; and/ or
	3. The drug was withdrawn and this made no difference to the event when clinically recovery would be expected. [This would not apply for some serious events such as myocardial infarction, or events causing permanent damage]; and / or
	It is strongly suggestive of a non-causal relationship if the drug was continued and the event resolved.
Unclassified (or, Conditional)	These are reports with insufficient data to establish a relationship and more data are expected. This is a temporary repository and the category for these events will be finalized when the new data become available.
Un-assessable	1. An event has occurred in association with a drug, but there are insufficient data to make an assessment.
	2. Some of the data may be contradictory or inconsistent.
	3. Details of the report cannot be supplemented or verified.

The WHO causality system is basically a combined assessment, taking into account the clinical-pharmacological aspects of the case history and the quality of documentation of observation, while prior knowledge of the ADR plays a less significant part.

Alert on WHO Causality Assessment:

- When there is no re-challenge or the outcome of re-challenge is unknown: Relationship cannot be termed CERTAIN.
- When there is no de-challenge or the outcome of de-challenge is unknown: Relationship cannot be termed PROBABLE.
- When the outcome of the event is unknown: relationship can be termed PROBABLE.
- When there are other possible causes of the event: relationship cannot be termed PROBABLE.

Naranjo probability scale (Algorithm): The Naranjo Probability Scale is another widely used scale for causality assessment. This uses questionnaires and points are added or taken away based on the response to each question. The total score is then used to decide the category as: definite, probable, possible or doubtful. It is helpful for assessing unexpected ADRs and useful for evaluators with little experience.

Questions	Yes	No	Don't Know	Categorization
1. Are there previous conclusive reports on this reaction?	+1	0	0	If the total score is more than 9, then certain; if the total score is between 5 – 8, then probable; if the total score is between 1 – 4, then possible and if the total score is 0 (zero), then unlikely.
2. Did the ADR appear after the suspected drug was administered?	+2	-1	0	
3. Did the ADR improve when the drug was discontinued or specific antagonist was administered?	+1	0	0	
4. Did the ADR reappear with re-challenge (administered again)?	+2	-1	0	
5. Are there alternative causes for the ADR (other than the drug) that could solely have caused the reaction?	-1	+2	0	
6. Did the reaction appear when placebo was given?	-1	+1	0	
7. Was the drug detected in blood (or other fluids) at toxic levels?	+1	0	0	
8. Was the reaction more severe when the dose was increased, or less severe when the dose was decreased?	+1	0	0	
9. Did the patient have a similar reaction to the same or similar drug in any previous exposure?	+1	0	0	
10. Was the ADR confirmed by any objective evidence?	+1	0	0	

Points to remember:

- The quality of data and documentation influence the reliability of the method. Often, individual systems of causality assessment are non-comparable.

- The relationship of a single report can be established but firm opinion may not be possible.

- A causality assessment is viewed as provisional and subject to change when new information or knowledge is made available.

- It is often unethical to re-challenge with the patients who experience severe haematological toxicities. Thus without a re-challenge, it is difficult to achieve causality rating of 'definite'.

***Preventability*:** Preventing Adverse Drug Reactions are not only possible but are necessary in both patient's and health system's interest. It has been reported that more than 50% adverse drug reactions may be preventable. Most ADRs are related to the prescribing of an incorrect dose or the administration of a drug to the patient with a known allergy.

There are several instruments/scales suggested for assessing the preventability of an ADR and they vary widely. However, they share the same basis for defining preventability. It seems Modified Schumock and Thornton scale is more acceptable. This scale divides preventability into three categories as: definitely preventable, probably preventable and not preventable.

Definitely Preventable	Parameters to be assessed	Comment
	1. Was there a history of allergy or previous reaction to the drug?	Answering YES to one or more of the parameters implies that ADR is definitely preventable. (If the answers are all NEGATIVE, proceed to next section given below)
	2. Was the drug involved inappropriate for the patient's clinical condition?	
	3. Was the dose, route or frequency of administration inappropriate for the patient's age, weight or disease state?	
Probably Preventable	1. Was the required therapeutic drug monitoring or other necessary laboratory tests not performed?	Answering YES to one or more of these parameters implies that ADR is probably preventable. [if answer are all NEGATIVE to these parameters, proceed to next section below]
	2. Was a documented drug interaction involved in the ADR?	
	3. Was poor compliance involved in the ADR?	
	4. Was a preventable measure not administered to the patient?	
	5. If a preventable measure was administered, was it inadequate or inappropriate? ANSWER NO IF THIS QUESTION IS NOT APPLICABLE.	
Not Preventable	If the ADR does not fall into the above two categories: definitely preventable or probably preventable.	

Preventing ADRs in Health Facilities Level: The following actions are advocated at health facility level to promote medicines' safety and help reducing occurrence of ADRs:

- Documenting the previous history of ADR of the patient.
- Introducing ADR reporting programme and encourage healthcare professionals to participate.
- Educating and sensitizing staff on need of ADRs through continuing professional development programme, through drug bulletins, and through reports of collected adverse events.
- Closely monitoring the high risk medicines.
- Closely monitoring high risk patients like pregnant women, breast feeding women, elderly persons, and persons with kidney or liver impairment.
- Reviewing the adverse reaction report on regular basis and updating the healthcare staff on incidence and impact of ADRs.
- Revise the medicine list and treatment guidelines in the light of significant ADRs.

Key Messages

- The adverse event reports are required to be evaluated for severity, probable causality and preventability.
- The severity of adverse drug reaction is classified as severe, moderate, mild and incidental.
- WHO scale and Naranjo probability scale are two widely accepted methods of causality assessment. WHO has six causality categories: certain (definite), probable, possible, unlikely, unclassified (or, conditional) and un-assessable (un-classifiable).
- Naranjo probability scale is based on the scoring system for a set of 10 questions: Score more than 9 means certain, score between 5 to 8 means probable, score between 1 to 4 means possible, and score 0 means unlikely.
- Modified Schumock and Thornton scale is an acceptable method for classifying preventability of adverse drug events: definitely preventable, probably preventable and not preventable.

Bibliography

1. A Practical Handbook on the Pharmacovigilance of Antiretroviral Medicines, World Health Organization, 2009.

2. Kathleen Holloway and Terry Green, Drug and Therapeutics Committees, A Practical Guide, World Health Organization and Management Sciences for Health, 2003.

3. K. G. Revikumar and B. D. Miglani, A Textbook of Pharmacy Practice, First Edition, Career Publications, 2009.

4. Ron Mann and Elizabeth Andrews (Ed), Pharmacovigilance, Second Edition, John Wiley & Sons Ltd, 2007.

5. SK Gupta (Ed), Textbook of Pharmacovigilance, First Edition, Jaypee Brothers Medical Publishers (P) Ltd., 2011.

Chapter 6

Signal: Identification and Strengthening

"I do not want two diseases: one nature made and one doctor made".

Napoleon Bonaparte

After reading this chapter, you should be able to understand and appreciate:
• Definition of Signal.
• Methods of Signal Identification.
• Evaluation of Signals (signal strengthening).
• WHO leadership in Signal Detection.

During clinical trials with limited time and limited exposure, all adverse effects are not identified. As some of the ADRs can be identified only after long exposure of the drug and to large population, the safety monitoring of the product continues after marketing approval. The primary objective of the safety monitoring of the medicine (also known as Pharmacovigilance) is the early detection of previously unknown adverse effects of the medicines. The early detection of the safety issues would help promoting safe use of medicines. The early warning sign is known as signal. Similarly in risk management process, identification of the possible hazard is the first step. After identifying the hazard, it is investigated further and if required, action is initiated to minimise the risk.

It is necessary to provide right environment for health professionals to be observant and critical in their diagnoses and therapy, so that they do not miss any piece of new information that may make therapy safer. The careful, informed, routine, systematic and standardised clinical review of reports of adverse drug events with the recording and appropriate collation of good data provides the quickest and justified way of identifying the previously unsuspected adverse reactions. It is important that safety of all medicines is monitored throughout their marketed life.

The World Health Organization defines Signal as "Reported information on a possible causal relationship between an adverse event and a drug, the relationship being unknown or incompletely documented previously."

The important points to remember are:

- The new information relevant to drug safety may come from different sources: reports of adverse events, clinical or non-clinical experiments, and published articles.

- Safety signal is suggestive of something new which would be worth further investigating. It is not confirmed safety issue.

- Newness may be on emerging trends and changes on specificity, severity, and/or rate of occurrence of a previously known adverse drug reaction. It may not be fully new.

- Safety signal precedes further investigation in determining whether or not a possible association rises to the level of warranting further action.

The continuing safety monitoring system should be available to: ensure regular screening of all sources of information to identify any potential signal; ensure appropriate action in response to new evidence that impacts on the known risk-benefit ratio; and communicate appropriately on risk-benefit changes to the drug regulating authority, healthcare professionals and the patients.

The following criteria are indicators for identifying events for investigation: good data; the event is clinically relevant; several reports showing credible and strong relationship with the drug (certain or probable); and the event would be significant if validated.

Spontaneous reporting of Adverse Events is the most common method used in Pharmacovigilance. It is helpful in detecting type B effects such as allergic or idiosyncratic reactions. The type B reactions occur only in minority of patients and usually unrelated to dosage and they are serious, unexplained and unpredictable too. Spontaneous reporting is also helpful in detecting unusual type A effects. The type A effects are pharmacologic effects of the drug and are dose related. Other sources of signal are: prescription event monitoring, large automated data resources on morbidity and drug use, case control surveillance and follow up studies. Type C effects (these effects related to an increased frequency of spontaneous disease) are difficult to study.

Methods of Signal Identification

I. *Clinical assessment of individual events*:

Careful, routine, standardised clinical assessment of individual reports with alertness to the possibility of a signal is the quickest method of detecting signal. The following points provide a guide to be adopted sequentially:

- When it is sensed to be a new type of adverse reaction, a search for records of similar events is warranted to confirm the opinion;
- The database needs to be checked for similar reports or clinically related terms;
- The adverse reaction should be checked in the reference source/s;
- If there is no reference of the occurrence of the event, investigation is needed to be continued.

A single report of a suspected adverse reaction can only rarely be considered as a signal itself. One can never be certain about a causal relationship between drug exposure and the adverse event on the basis of one individual case. It is only through on-going analysis of the collection of events that a potential signal is generated.

II. *Systematic review of multiple case reports*:All the events in the database for the drug(s) of interest are to be reviewed at regular intervals. The periodicity of the systemic review of cumulative data for the purpose of signal detection depends on the amount of safety data received or available in the database. One month frequency may be acceptable.

There are various methods for review of data as a part of signal detection, ranging from manual review of individual cases to the use of computer algorithms of drug safety database (also known as data mining). Every method has its own advantages and disadvantages. Individual case review allows complete evaluation of every aspect of the case but often is an issue of resource constraint. Simple counts of number of suspected adverse reactions or a frequency analysis can highlight the appearance of a new reaction or an increase in the occurrence of a known reaction. It is necessary to consider at what point an increase in number or frequency of a suspected adverse reaction becomes significant. Is the increase due to increase in sales?

III. *Record linkage*:

Literally the record linkage is the systematic bringing together of the records of the individuals in a large population. In Pharmacovigilance, record linkage is the linkage of patient specific information that is stored separately.

The record linkage is possible on the availability of a unique identifier for the patients either in the health system or in hospital record. This same identifier must be recorded with the patient details in the cohort database. The process involves matching the details in cohort database with that of hospital or other records. This would enable to see the details of the patient: whether the patient died and the cause of death; whether patient was admitted to hospital and the diagnosis etc. The review result is recorded in the patient's database in cohort.

An unexpectedly high rate of a particular event like liver damage may represent a signal.

IV. *Automated signal detection*:

The automated statistical methods used in the analysis of safety data include the proportional reporting ratio (PRR). PRR is a method that uses software to measure the proportion of reports in the database with a particular drug – event combination and compares this proportion with that for the same event in the reports for all other drugs combined. This requires a large set of data and exceptionally high reporting of suspected adverse reaction of one type or in one system organ class. If the PRR for a particular drug –event combination is significantly high, and it is not a recognised reaction, it may represent a signal. PRR methods are somewhat experimental and they lack reliability.

Though earlier PRR system was used by both pharmaceutical companies and the regulatory authorities, the system is being replaced by empirical Bayesian methods. While it is beyond the scope of this text giving more details of Bayesian methods, a brief description is given. The commonly used Bayesian methods include: The Bayesian Confidence Propagation Neural Network (BCPNN) and Multi – Item Gamma Poisson Shrinker (MGPS), for the purpose of signal detection. Medicines and Healthcare Products Regulatory Agency (MHRA) of UK employs MGPS and Uppsala Monitoring Centre (UMC) uses BCPNN (and data mining) techniques for signal detection.

All signals identified from statistical programmes require subsequent clinical evaluation.

V. *Other sources of information*:

The responsible professional should look into the periodic safety update reports, information from new non-clinical research, post marketing studies, clinical trials and from other initiatives such as surveys and registries. The few good sources too can be explored for information on ADRs: Martindale's The Complete Drug Reference, The Physician's Desk Reference, and Micromedex online drug reference etc.

If there is no good evidence of an event being recognised as an adverse reaction in two – or more of these references and if warranted clinically, it should be investigated further as a possible signal.

Signal Detection Algorithms (SDAs): They have been accepted as the vital tools used with reasonable predictive accuracy in signalling adverse events. For identifying safety signals of adverse events from spontaneous reports, data mining techniques are increasingly used to supplement the traditional expert review of reports and to analyse the large volume of accumulated data more rapidly. These data mining techniques are known as SDAs.

The SDAs are the tools used to analyse the databases of spontaneous reports for concealed associations between drugs and reported adverse events that may evade the scrutiny of manual assessment. SDAs are designed to compute surrogate measures of statistical association between drug-event pairs reported in a database. These measures are often interpreted as signal scores, with larger values representing stronger associations indicating more likely to represent true ADRs. The regulatory bodies like USFDA regularly uses SDAs to the Adverse Events Reports in order to monitor, prioritise, and identify new safety signals of Adverse Drug Events that require further investigation.

Signal Detection Method Used by Pharmacovigilance Programme of India: Following parameters are considered:

Parameters	Threshold Value	Comment
Information Component (IC)	$IC_{025} > 0$	Fulfilment of at least two of these four parameters is required for considering a specific drug-ADR combination as a potential signal.
Proportional Relative Risk / Proportional Reporting Ratio (PRO)	PRR ≥ 2 with the lower bound of its 95% CI > 1	
Chi-square ($\chi 2$) statistics (with 1 degree of freedom)	$\chi 2$ statistics (with 1 degree of freedom) ≥ 4	IC_{025} is the lower limit of the 95% highest posterior density interval of the IC.
Total number of reports on the specific Drug-ADR combination available in the Indian database (Ncomb)	Ncomb ≥ 3, to highlight potential signals	

Signal strengthening: The potential signals generally require further investigation for making a decision whether the product in question caused the event. It is necessary to perform a review of the case(s) that prompted the initial signal alert in addition to performing a search for any additional cases and other information relevant to the issue. The clinical evaluation of identified signals is called strengthening of signals. The indepth review of the cases is usually based on the following principles:

(i) Reviewing other experience: Look for the all available data source for similar reports. While performing searches, the search terms are carefully selected to ensure all relevant cases are retrieved;

(ii) Searching for non-random patterns: Examination of data on a group of reports may show patterns that are not random, and in the absence of biases, non-random pattern suggest that the event may be related to the medicine. Example –when compared with the cohort, if the rate of events in women and men are significantly different, then drug effect could be one of the reasons;

(iii) Reviewing the pharmacology: To find out whether there is any plausible mechanism by which the medicine could cause the event;

(iv) Consulting expert safety review panel and other experts – The reviewers are asked to review the case reports using their clinical experience and pharmacological knowledge;

(v) Undertaking epidemiological studies: The following studies may be essential: cohort studies, case control studies, record linkage studies, and population database studies;

(vi) Communicating to stakeholders: Effective and well presented communication of the signal to all stakeholders seeking their feedback would help validating the signal. The following stakeholders may be considered seeking their opinion: expert safety review panel, regulatory authority, health professionals, pharmaceutical company, Uppsala Monitoring ADR bulletin and medical journals.

World Health Organization's Leadership in Signal Detection: WHO programme for International Drug Monitoring is managed by its collaborating centre, the Uppsala Drug Monitoring Centre. The UMC team regularly searches Vigibase for new signals and communicates the results to the regulatory authorities of member countries. Vigibase is the name for the WHO International ADR database. UMC uses Bayesian Confidence Propagation Neural Network [BCPNN] technique for finding new drug-ADR combinations likely to be signals through quantitative filtering of the data. This focuses clinical review on the potentially most important combinations of drugs and adverse drug reactions. Other useful information can also be obtained from Vigibase such as variation in ADR patterns in different countries. The causes of such differences may be due to different ingredients in the formulation, different dosage or different indications for use.

The Review Process: The data in Vigibase is scanned using automated data mining programme, the BCPNN, to produce a database with case information and occurrence of drug – ADRs including a content table. The results are presented in a computerised table called **Combination Database**. At this stage the list is neither filtered nor analyzed or reviewed. The list is sent periodically to the National centres who review its international contents for issue of relevance to their own country.

Based on statistical threshold and the Information Component (IC) values the promising drug-ADR pairs are copied into **Association Database**. They are considered worth examining further. The IC values for drug – event combinations can be plotted as graphs over time to examine any trend. A positive signal will have IC values that become more significant over time as more cases are included.

A filtering process is applied to narrow down the number of combinations for review and to focus on the areas of the greatest importance. This is to establish a priority focus through predefined algorithms which may also consider: rapid reporting increase, serious reaction and new drug, special interest reactions, to give a manageable number of combinations.

Contd...

Then the prioritised drug – ADR combinations are checked for their occurrence in the available literatures such Martindale's Complete Drug Reference, Physician's Drug Reference, DrugDex etc., to see what is known and whether the combinations have merits to pass to reviewers for indepth study. For drugs where the reaction is not available in the literature or not fully described, it is necessary to retrieve the complete case reports from Vigibase. These are then sent to appropriate expert in the review panel with a request to assess the evidence for the relationship of the reaction to the suspected drug. The material for review is divided into System Organ Classes (SOC) for the ADRs and Anatomical, Therapeutic, Chemical (ATC) Groups for the drugs.

The International experts drawn from different countries are requested to assess the case reports using their clinical experience and pharmacological knowledge. Analysis of potential signals includes checking the available case data and making literature searches. After assessing the cases, including the judgement on the causal strength of the drug –ADR association, the reviewer drafts a short report on the signal if felt worth notifying to the National centres. After review within the UMC, the text of the report is included in SIGNAL for distribution to National Centres. SIGNAL is the restricted publication of UMC.

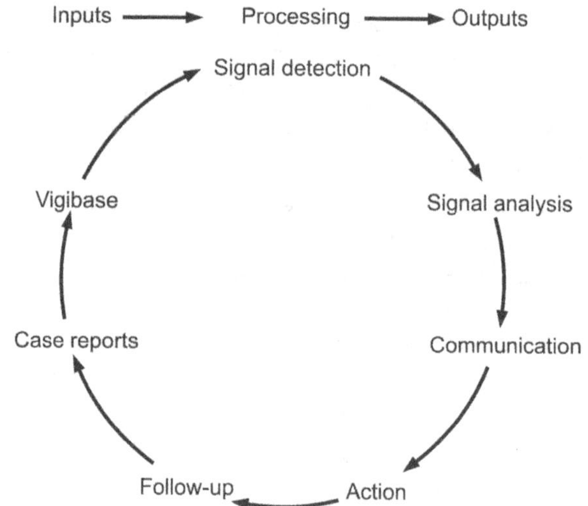

Source: View Point, Part 2, the Uppsala Monitoring Centre, 2004.

Fig. 6.1: Flow Chart Showing the Principal Elements of the Pharmacovigilance at the International Level [From Report to Final]

While it is not possible to have equally effective Pharmacovigilance programme in every country, WHO's International database provides enough information on safety issues to the regulatory authorities and pharmaceutical companies, of resource constrained countries, to take appropriate action reducing medicine use related harms.

[Source: View Point – Part 2, *the* Uppsala Monitoring Centre, 2004.]

Investigation of signals is an iterative process and at each stage there should be consideration of the need for communication with regulatory authorities and /or implementation of risk minimisation measures. When a new signal is identified, it is important to consider the potential of increased risk and change in its risk – benefit. The pharmaceutical companies should notify the regulatory authority immediately of any change in the balance of risks and benefits of their products. Upon confirmation of new signal for a product, the following action may be initiated:

- Variation of the summary of product characteristics or product information leaflets;

- Provision of safety information directly to healthcare professionals and public.

It must be remembered that the pharmaceutical companies must not communicate to the healthcare professionals or patients without approval of the regulatory authorities.

VigiRank- a novel method for signal detection: VigiRank is recently developed by UMC to screen database of individual case reports for possible new safety signals with medicines. While the usual screening relied on disproportionality analysis which is based on aggregate number of reports, the new VigiRank incorporates disproportionate reporting as just one component. In addition, VigiRank considers several aspects related to the quality and the contents of the reports. The new method simultaneously considers the number of informative reports, recent reports, and reports with free text description, as well as geographical spread of reporting. It is believed, at this stage of writing this text, VigiRank would help uncover signals that would be missed by disproportionality analysis alone and reduce the number of false leads.

[Uppsala Reports October 2014]

Key Messages

- One of the most important aspects of drug – safety monitoring of marketed products is the identification and analysis of new, medically important findings that might influence the use of medicines.

- Serious signals that appear to be new and relate to new drugs usually elicit regulatory action. Less serious signals though have significant morbidity or compliance, may not be investigated so vigorously even when the numbers build up.

Contd...

- The factors that determine the evidence contained in a signal: quantitative strength of association, consistency of the data, exposure response relationship, biological plausibility, experimental findings, possible analysis, and the nature and quality of data.

- The BCPNN runs on all reported events worldwide and therefore, there are greater chances of finding more reports of the suspect drug – event combination.

- The WHO programme usually considers signals if they are involved in more than one country.

Bibliography

1. A Practical Handbook on the Pharmacovigilance of Antiretroviral Medicines, World Health Organization, 2009.

2. Atsuko Shibata and Manfred Hauben, Pharmacovigilance, Signal Detection and Signal Intelligence Review, 14th International Conference on Information Fusion, Chicago, USA, 2011.

3. Guideline on Good Pharmacovigilance Practices, Module IX-Signal Management, European Medicines Agency, 22 June 2012.

4. Patrick Waller, An introduction to Pharmacovigilance, Wiley –Blackwell, 2010.

5. Ronald HB Meyboom *et al*, Principles of Signal Detection in Pharmacovigilance, Drug Safety, 16(6), June 1997.

Chapter 7

Quality Assurance in Pharmacovigilance

"Fortunately a surgeon who uses the wrong side of the scalpel cuts his own fingers and not the patient's; if the same applied to drugs, they would have investigated very carefully a long time ago".

Rudolph Bucheim
Beitrage Zur Arzneimitteellehre (1849)

After reading this chapter, you should be able to understand and appreciate:
• Concept of quality assurance and quality control in Pharmacovigilance system;
• Concept of Good Pharmacovigilance;
• Quality Assurance Process in Pharmacovigilance; and
• Indicators which may be used to assess a pharmacovigilance system.

In a quality conscious world, the pharmacovigilance system needs to ensure that the key activities and processes are being performed in accordance with expected procedures promoting good pharmacovigilance practice. There are two main stakeholders: National Medicine Regulatory Authority and Marketing Authorization Holders who are responsible for ensuring the functioning of quality system in pharmacovigilance activities.

The quality management system aims to build the quality to the product or process through planned and systematic activities. There are four important components in a quality management system: quality planning, quality control programme, quality assurance and quality improvement. The quality planning defines the quality criteria and provides the resources. The quality control programme provides the means to monitor and check the result of the process against the quality parameters. Quality control is the observation techniques and activities that are used to fulfil requirements for quality. Quality assurance is the planned and systematic activities in a quality system so that the quality requirement for a programme or system is ensured. Quality assurance is achieved through continuous evaluation of quality control activities at every step in the process and implementing the corrective measures. Quality improvement provides opportunity for improving the system based on experience and feedback. Unanticipated problems can be redressed through quality management system.

Good Pharmacovigilance Practices (GPvP) are set of measures required to facilitate the performance of pharmacovigilance system. A quality system in place would ensure good pharmacovigilance practices. GPvP guidelines describe how to establish a quality system in pharmacovigilance to ensure quality. GPvP is based on acquiring complete data from spontaneous adverse event reports (also called case reports). A good report should have at least the following elements:

- Description of adverse events;
- Details of suspected drug and concomitant drug therapy;
- Patient details;
- Details of diagnosis of events;
- Therapeutic measures and laboratory data at base line, during therapy and subsequent to therapy; and
- Details of de-challenge or re-challenge.

The regulatory authorities of US, UK etc., have issued GPvP guidance documents for adoption by pharmaceutical industries.

While it is beyond the scope of this chapter to discuss all aspects of quality system, three important issues are discussed: quality issues of data, audit programme of activities and assessing the programme.

I. *Quality of Data*:

In spite of introduction of active pharmacovigilance activities, the spontaneous reporting continues to be the main data source for pharmacovigilance activities. The whole process of data collection to retrieval and analysis must have rigorous procedure to ensure the best possible quality data. The management of data is also equally important.

There must be formal process and procedure [Standard Operating Procedure] in place to ensure the accuracy and completeness of the data. Data quality is based on/assessed by consistency in contents and nomenclature, level of details, data entry process, accuracy, relevance and completeness. .

II. *Pharmacovigilance Audit*:

Pharmacovigilance audit activities meant to verify, by examination and evaluation of objective evidence, the appropriateness and effectiveness of the implementation and operation of a pharmacovigilance system, including its quality system for pharmacovigilance activities.

In general, an audit is a systematic, disciplined, independent and documented process for obtaining evidence and evaluating the evidence objectively to determine the extent to which the audit criteria are fulfilled, contributing to the improvement of risk management, control and governance processes. Audit evidence consists of records, statements or other information, which are relevant to the audit criteria and verifiable. Audit criteria are, for each audit objective, the standards of performance and control against which the auditee and its activities will be assessed. In the context of pharmacovigilance, audit criteria should reflect the requirements for the pharmacovigilance system, including its quality system for pharmacovigilance activities, as found in the legislation and guidance.

A. The risk-based approach to pharmacovigilance audits

A risk-based approach is one that uses techniques to determine the areas of risk, where risk is defined as the probability of an event occurring that will have an impact on the achievement of objectives, taking account of the severity of its outcome and/or likelihood of non-detection by other methods. The risk-based approach to audits focuses on the areas of highest risk to the organisation's pharmacovigilance system, including its quality system for pharmacovigilance activities. In the context of pharmacovigilance, the risk to public health is of prime importance. Risk can be assessed at the following stages:

- Long term audit planning resulting in an audit strategy (long term approach), which should be endorsed by upper management;

- Short term audit planning resulting in an audit programme, setting audit objectives, and the extent and boundaries, often termed as scope, of the audits in that programme; and

- Operational level audit planning resulting in an audit plan for individual audit engagements, prioritising audit tasks based on risk and utilising risk-based sampling and testing approaches, and reporting of audit findings in line with their relative risk level and audit recommendations in line with the suggested grading system

Risk assessment should be documented appropriately for the long term, short term and operational planning of pharmacovigilance audit activity in the organisation

(a) *Long term audit planning*: A high level statement of how the audit activities will be delivered over a period of time, longer than the annual programme, usually for a period of 2-5 years. The audit strategy includes a list of audits that could reasonably be performed. The audit strategy is used to outline the areas highlighted for audit, the audit topics as well as the methods and assumptions (including e.g., risk assessment) on which the audit programme is based.

The audit strategy should cover the governance, risk management and internal controls of all parts of the pharmacovigilance system including:

- All pharmacovigilance processes and tasks;

- The quality system for pharmacovigilance activities;

- Interactions and interfaces with other departments, as appropriate;

- Pharmacovigilance activities conducted by affiliated organisations or activities delegated to another organisation (e.g., regional reporting centres, MAH affiliates or third parties, such as contract organisations and other vendors).

This is a non-prioritised, non-exhaustive list of examples of risk factors that could be considered for the purposes of a risk assessment:

- Changes to legislation and guidance;

- Major re-organisation or other re-structuring of the pharmacovigilance system, mergers, acquisitions (specifically for marketing authorisation holders, this may lead to a significant increase in the number of products for which the system is used);

- Change in key managerial function(s);
- Risk to availability of adequately trained and experienced pharmacovigilance staff, e.g. due to significant turn-over of staff, deficiencies in training processes, re-organisation, increase in volumes of work;
- Significant changes to the system since the time of a previous audit, e.g. introduction of a new database(s) for pharmacovigilance activities or of a significant upgrade to the existing database(s), changes to processes and activities in order to address new or amended regulatory requirements;
- First medicinal product on the market (for a marketing authorisation holder);
- Medicinal product(s) on the market with specific risk minimisation measures or other specific safety conditions such as requirements for additional monitoring;
- Criticality of the process, e.g.,how critical is the area/process to proper functioning of the pharmaco-vigilance system. When deciding when to audit an affiliate or third party, the marketing authorisation holder should consider the nature and criticality of the pharmacovigilance activities that are being performed by an affiliate or third party on behalf of the marketing authorisation holder, in addition to considering the other factors included in this list;

Outcome of previous audits, e.g., has the area/process ever been audited (if not, then this may need to be prioritised depending on criticality); if the area/process has previously been audited, the audit findings* are a factor to consider when deciding when to re-audit the area/process, including the implementation of agreed actions;

- Identified procedural gaps relating to specific areas/processes;
- Other organisational changes that could negatively impact on the area/process, e.g., if a change occurs to a

support function (such as information technology support) this could negatively impact upon pharmacovigilance activities.

(b) ***Short term audit planning***: An audit programme is a set of one or more audits planned for a specific timeframe, normally for a year. It should be prepared in line with the long term audit strategy. The audit programme should be approved by upper management with overall responsibility for operational and governance structure.

The risk-based audit programme should be based on an appropriate risk assessment and should focus on:

- The quality system for pharmacovigilance activities;
- Critical pharmacovigilance processes;
- Key control systems relied on for pharmacovigilance activities;
- Areas identified as high risk, after controls have been put in place or mitigating action taken.

The risk-based audit programme should also take into account historical areas with insufficient past audit coverage, and high risk areas identified by and/or specific requests from management and/or persons responsible for pharmacovigilance activities.

The audit programme documentation should include a brief description of the plan for each audit to be delivered, including an outline of scope and objectives.

The rationale for the timing, periodicity and scope of the individual audits which form part of the audit programme should be based on the documented risk assessment. However, risk-based pharmacovigilance audit(s) should be performed at regular intervals, which are in line with legislative requirements.

Changes to the audit programme may happen and will require proper documentation.

(c) ***Operational level audit planning and reporting***

    (i) ***Planning and fieldwork***: The organisation should ensure that written procedures are in place regarding the planning and conduct of individual audits that will be delivered. Timeframes for all the steps required for the performance of an individual audit should be settled in the relevant audit related procedures, and the organisation should ensure that audits are conducted in accordance with the written procedures, in line with applicable regulation of that country.

Individual pharmacovigilance audits should be undertaken in line with the approved risk-based audit programme. When planning individual audits, the auditor identifies and assesses the risks relevant to the area under review and employs the most appropriate risk-based sampling and testing methods, documenting the audit approach in an audit plan.

(ii) *Audit reporting*: The findings of the auditors should be documented in an audit report and should be communicated to management in a timely manner. The audit process should include mechanisms for communicating the audit findings to the auditee and receiving feedback, and reporting the audit findings to management and relevant parties, including those responsible for pharmacovigilance systems, in accordance with legal requirements and guidance on pharmacovigilance audits. Audit findings should be reported in line with their relative risk level and should be graded in order to indicate their relative criticality to risks impacting the pharmacovigilance system, processes and parts of processes. The grading system should be defined in the description of the quality system for pharmacovigilance, and should take into consideration the thresholds noted below which would be used in further reporting:

- *Critical* is a fundamental weakness in one or more pharmacovigilance processes or practices that adversely affects the whole pharmacovigilance system and/or the rights, safety or well-being of patients, or that poses a potential risk to public health and/or represents a serious violation of applicable regulatory requirements.

- *Major* is a significant weakness in one or more pharmacovigilance processes or practices, or a fundamental weakness in part of one or more pharmacovigilance processes or practices that is detrimental to the whole process and/or could potentially adversely affect the rights, safety or well-being of patients and/or could potentially pose a risk to public health and/or represents a violation of applicable regulatory requirements which is however not considered serious.

- *Minor* is a weakness in the part of one or more pharmacovigilance processes or practices that is not expected to adversely affect the whole pharmacovigilance system or process and/or the rights, safety or well-being of patients.

  Issues that need to be urgently addressed should be communicated in an expedited manner to the auditee's management and the upper management.

(iii) *Actions based on audit outcomes and follow-up of audits:*

Actions: immediate action, prompt action, action within a reasonable timeframe, issues that need to be urgently addressed, or communicated in an expedited manner, are intended to convey timelines that are appropriate, relevant, and in line with the relative risk to the pharmacovigilance system.

Corrective and preventive actions to address critical and major issues should be prioritised. The precise timeframe for action(s) related to a given critical finding, for example, may differ depending on nature of findings and the planned action(s).

The management of the organisation is responsible for ensuring that the organisation has a mechanism in place to adequately address the issues arising from pharmacovigilance audits. Actions should include root cause analysis and impact analysis of identified audit findings and preparation of a corrective and preventive action plan, where appropriate.

Upper management and those charged with governance, should ensure that effective action is implemented to address the audit findings. The implementation of agreed actions should be monitored in a systematic way, and the progress of implementation should be communicated on a periodic basis proportionate to the planned actions to upper management.

Evidence of completion of actions should be recorded in order to document that issues raised during the audit have been addressed.

Capacity for follow-up audits should be foreseen in the audit programme. They should be carried out as deemed necessary, in order to verify the completion of agreed actions.

(iv) ***Quality system and record management practices:***

The organisation should assign the specific responsibilities for the pharmacovigilance audit activities. Pharmacovigilance audit activities should be independent. The organisation's management should ensure this independence and objectivity in a structured manner and document this.

Auditors should be free from interference in determining the scope of auditing, performing pharmacovigilance audits and communicating audit results. The main reporting line should be to the upper management with overall responsibility for operational and governance structure that allows the auditor(s) to fulfil their responsibilities and to provide independent, objective audit opinion. Auditors can consult with technical experts, personnel involved in pharmacovigilance processes, and with the person responsible for pharmacovigilance; however auditors should maintain an unbiased attitude that allows them to perform audit work in such a manner that they have an honest belief in their work product and that no significant quality compromises are made. Objectivity requires auditors not to subordinate their judgement on audit matters to that of others.

(v) ***Qualifications, skills and experience of auditors and continuing professional development:*** Auditors should demonstrate and maintain proficiency in terms of the knowledge, skills and abilities required to effectively conduct and/or participate in pharmacovigilance audit activities. The proficiency of audit team members will have been gained through a combination of education, work experience and training and, as a team, should cover knowledge, skills and abilities in:

- Audit principles, procedures and techniques;
- Applicable laws, regulations and other requirements relevant to pharmacovigilance;
- Pharmacovigilance activities, processes and system(s);
- Management system(s);
- Organisational system(s).

(vi) *Evaluation of the quality of audit activities:*Evaluation of audit work can be undertaken by means of ongoing and periodic assessment of all audit activities, auditee feedback and self-assessment of audit activities (e.g., quality assurance of audit activities, compliance to code of conduct, audit programme, and audit procedures).

(vii) *Audits undertaken by outsourced audit service providers:* Ultimate responsibility for the operation and effectiveness of the pharmacovigilance system resides within the organisation. Where the organisation decides to use an outsourced audit service provider to implement the pharmacovigilance audit requirements on the basis of applicable regulation and perform pharmacovigilance audits:

- The requirements and preparation of the audit risk assessment, the audit strategy and audit programme and individual engagements should be specified to the outsourced service providers, by the organisation, in writing;
- The scope, objectives and procedural requirements for the audit should be specified to the outsourced service provider, by the organisation, in writing;
- The organisation should obtain and document assurance of the independence and objectivity of outsourced service providers;
- The outsourced audit service provider should also follow the relevant regulatory requirement.

III. *Assessment of Pharmacovigilance System*:

It is always necessary to assess a system in order to ensure that the system functions in the expected way. The evaluation of data collection practice, analysis of data and interpretation of data at different level of the system would help develop recommendations and identify priority interventions to improve the critical aspects of pharmacovigilance system. The outcome of a pharmacovigilance system should be reduction in medicine related problems. Management Sciences for Health, USA, has developed 43 indicators that address the following five components:

(a) Policy, law and regulation;

(b) Systems, structures, and stake holders coordination;

(c) Signal generation and data management;

(d) Risk assessment and evaluation; and

(e) Risk management and communication.

There are 26 core indicators and 17 supplementary indicators. Core indictors are important and essential. The core indicators with their importance are given in the table given below. The readers are encouraged to refer the original publication to learn about the supplementary indictors.

S. No.	Indicator	What for Used	Frequency of Assessment
	Policy, Law and Regulation		
1	Existence of a policy document that contains essential statements on pharmacovigilance (stand alone or as a part of some other policy document)	Structural	Every five years
2	Existence of specific legal provisions for pharmacovigilance in the national medicines legislation or similar legislation	Structural	Every five years
	Systems, Structures, and Stakeholder Coordination		
3	Existence of a pharmacovigilance center or unit	Structural	Every five years
4	Pharmacovigilance center or unit has a clear mandate, structure, roles, and responsibilities	Structural	Every five years

Contd...

S. No.	Indicator	What for Used	Frequency of Assessment
5	Existence of a medicine information or pharmacovigilance service that provides ADR and drug safety–related question-and-answer services	Structural	Annually
6	A designated staff responsible for pharmacovigilance or medicine safety activities	Structural	Annually
7	Dedicated budget available for pharmacovigilance-related activities	Structural	Annually
8	Existence of a national medicine safety advisory committee or a subcommittee with similar functions that has met at least once in the last year	Structural	Annually
9	Existence of national pharmacovigilance guidelines updated within the last five years	Structural	Every five years
10	Existence of protocols or SOPs for improving patient safety relating to medicine use	Structural	Annually
11	Existence of a minimum core list of communication technologies to improve access to safety reporting and provision of medicine information	Structural	Annually
12	Existence of an ADR or medicine safety bulletin (or any other health-related newsletter that routinely features ADR or medicine safety issues) published in the last six months	Structural	Annually
13	Platform or strategy exists for the coordination of pharmacovigilance activities at the national level	Structural	Annually
Signal Generation and Data Management			
14	Existence of a system for coordination and collation of pharmacovigilance data from all sources in the country (e.g., health programs, immunization program, active surveillance studies)	Process	Annually
15	Existence of a database for tracking pharmacovigilance activities	Process	Annually

Contd...

S. No.	Indicator	What for Used	Frequency of Assessment
16	Existence of a form for reporting suspected ADRs	Process	Annually
17	Existence of a form for reporting suspected product quality issues (as a subset in the ADR form or as a separate form)	Process	Annually
18	Existence of a form for reporting suspected medication errors (as a subset in the ADR form or as a separate form)	Process	Annually
19	Existence of a form for reporting suspected treatment failure (as a subset in the ADR form or as a separate form)	Process	Annually
Risk Assessment and Evaluation			
20	Number of ADR reports received in the last year	Process	Annually
21	Number of active surveillance activities currently ongoing or carried out in the last five years	Process	Every five years
22	Percentage of patients in public health programs for whom drug-related adverse events were reported in the last year (disaggregated by type of adverse event, drug, severity, outcomes, and demographics)	Process	Annually
23	Percentage of patients under going treatment within a public health program whose treatment was modified because of treatment failure or ADRs in the last year (disaggregated by treatment failure and ADRs)	Process	Annually
Risk Management and Communication			
24	Average time lag between identification of safety signal of a serious ADR or significant medicine safety issue and communication to health care workers and the public	Outcome	Annually

Contd...

S. No.	Indicator	What for Used	Frequency of Assessment
25	Percentage of the sampled Drug and Therapeutics Committees that have carried out pharmacovigilance activities or addressed medicine safety issues in the last year	Outcome	Annually
26	Percentage of medicines sampled in the last year that passed product quality tests	Outcome	Annually

The national medicine regulatory authority, public health programmes, health facilities and researchers concerned with pharmacovigilance can utilize these tools to assess the various segments of pharmacovigilance systems: structure, process and outcome.

Key Messages

- Quality control is the observation techniques and activities that are used to fulfil requirements for quality. Quality assurance is the planned and systematic activities implemented in a quality system to ensure quality requirements in a product or process. In general, quality assurance defines the standards to be followed in order to meet the requirements while quality control ensures that these standards are followed at every step.

- Good Pharmacovigilance Practices (GPvP) are set of measures required to facilitate the performance of pharmacovigilance system. A quality system in place would ensure good pharmacovigilance practices.

- Three important components of quality system: quality of data, auditing and periodic assessment of the programme.

- Quality of data focuses on good case report.

- Auditing verifies, through objective evidence, the appropriateness and effectiveness of the implementation and operation of a pharmacovigilance system including its quality system for pharmacovigilance activities.

- The evaluation of data collection practice, analysis of data and interpretation of data at different level of the system would help develop recommendations and identify priority interventions to improve the critical aspects of pharmacovigilance system. The indictor based assessment facilitates evaluation.

Bibliography

1. Guideline on good pharmacovigilance practices, EMA/541760/2011 Dated 22 June 2012, European Medicine Agency.

2. Indicator Based Pharmacovigilance Assessment Tool: Manual for Conducting Assessments in Developing Countries, Management Sciences for Health, December 2009.

3. Marie Lindquist, Data Quality Management in Pharmacovigilance, Drug Safety, 27(12), 2004.

4. WHO pharmacovigilance indicators, A practical manual for the assessment of pharmacovigilance system, World Health Organization, 2015.

[Contributed by Mr. Shaikh Ruhu Al Amin]

Chapter 8

Periodic Safety Update Reports

"The death of one man is a tragedy. The death of millions is a statistic".

Joe Stalin, comment to
Churchill at Potsdam, 1945

After reading this chapter, you should be able to understand and appreciate:
• Concept of Periodic Safety Update Reports [PSURs];
• Components of PSURs;
• How to develop PSURs and
• PSURs provisions of India, UK and USA.

Many medicinal/pharmaceutical products have been withdrawn from various markets over the years because of actual or perceived safety issues. It is estimated that one-third of them were withdrawn within two years of launch and half within five years. Withdrawal of products after marketing approval substantiate the need of submission of post marketing surveillance report of all approved drugs to the medicine regulatory authorities. The clinical trials in limited number of patients and in controlled condition cannot detect all possible adverse drug reactions. Many new adverse drug reactions are detected when drugs are in use in real world: large population, different co-morbid conditions and along with other drugs. Hence, the regulatory authorities throughout the world require that the marketing authorization holder (pharmaceutical company marketing the medicinal product) needs submitting the safety report periodically after marketing approval. This requirement is also known as post marketing surveillance. The submission of safety update reports periodically is called Periodic Safety Update Reports (PSURs).

The PSURs are defined as systematic review of global safety data which became available to the marketing authorization holder of a marketed medicinal product at predefined time interval. The purpose of the PSURs is to provide a comprehensive and critical analysis of risk-benefit balance of a medicinal product taking into account of new or emerging information in the cumulative risk-benefit analysis. The frequency of submission of the PSURs is usually mentioned in the marketing authorization. In general routine PSURs are not required for products of low risks like well established medicinal products and generics.

There are two main stake holders on PSUR: the companies who develop the PSUR and submit to the Regulatory Authority; and the Regulatory Authority who reviews the report and take regulatory decision. PSURs provide opportunities for the marketing authorization holder to review the safety profile of their products and ensure that summary of product characteristics and patient information leaflets are up to date. On the other hand, the quality of PSURs is a good indicator of overall state of Pharmacovigilance system of marketing authorization holders. For drug regulatory authorities, PSURs are valuable Pharmacovigilance data   to initiate regulatory decisions including banning a product.

In general PSUR begins with approval of medicinal product and continues for the entire marketing life of the product.

Periodicity: PSURs are not cumulative documents. They cover a predefined period which is specified by the regulatory authority. The frequency or periodicity varies from country to country. In European Union, the requirements are: six monthly PSURs for first two years, annual reports for next two years, and then five years report thereafter. In Japan, PSUR requirement for new chemical entity is every six months for two years and annually for next four years. For new formulation, PSUR is required for every six months for two years and then annually for next two years.

Content and format: Worldwide there are attempts to simplify the procedure as well as to make uniform format for submission of PSURs. The following is the basic structure of a PSUR:

- Executive Summary
- Introduction or scope of the report

- Worldwide marketing authorization status
- Action taken for safety reason and changes to core safety information
- Patient exposure data
- Individual case histories
- Information from formal studies
- Overall safety evaluation [important and newly identified or ongoing safety issues are documented and proposals to address them]
- Important information received after the data lock period (cut off date) or last report
- Core safety information

Each product is usually assigned an international birth date (IBD), the day of first approval anywhere in the world. This is the basis of cut off dates for submission of reports.

The readers are encouraged to see the prototype reports in Current Challenges in Pharmacovigilance: Pragmatic Approaches, Report of CIOMS working V, Geneva 2001 [http://www.cioms.ch/index.php/component/booklibrary/?task=view&Ite mid=&id=47&catid=58].

PSUR in India: Indian regulation [New Drugs and Clinical Trials Rules, 2019] requires that PSURs of new drugs are required to be submitted to the office of DCG (I) every six months for the first two years and thereafter annually for next two years. The PSURs due for the period must be submitted within 30 calendar days of the last day of the report. The manufacturers or importers are responsible for complying with this legal obligation.

The report should be India specific and must be structured to contain the followings:

1. A title page stating: Periodic Safety Update Report for the product, applicants name, period covered by the report, date of approval of the new drug, approved indication, date of marketing of new drug and date of reporting;
2. Introduction;
3. Current worldwide market authorization status;
4. Update of action taken for safety reasons;
5. Changes to reference safety information;

6. Estimated patient exposure;
7. Presentation of individual case histories;
8. Studies;
9. Other Information;
10. Overall safety evaluation;
11. Conclusion; and
12. Appendix providing material relating to indications, dosing, pharmacology and other related information.

Though PSURs are mandatory, the pharmaceutical companies do not comply with this requirement. This is evident from the report of Parliamentary Standing Committee on Health and Family Welfare [59th Report on Functioning of CDSCO, 2012]. The Committee observed that there was not only non-compliance on submission of reports but also the reports were neither India specific nor in appropriate format. The Committee strongly recommended the Ministry to warn the manufacturers of new drugs to comply with mandatory provision of PSURs or face suspension of marketing approval.

The Government of India now proposes to direct the pharmaceutical companies to have pharmacovigilance system to periodically submit safety update reports to the CDSCO, the central regulatory agency on Drugs and Medical Devices. The National Coordinating Centre of Pharmacovigilance Programme of India, Indian Pharmacopoeia Commission, too plans to set up dedicated cell to start work on reviewing the PSURs as Government plans to link PSURs to Pharmacovigilance Programme.

PSUR in USA: US FDA issued new guideline titled "Providing post-market periodic safety reports in the ICH E2C (R2) format [Periodic Benefit – Risk Evaluation Report (PBRER)]". PBRER replaced the earlier format of submitting PSURs as Periodic Adverse Drug Experience Report (PADER) or Periodic Adverse Experience Report (PAER) or PSUR. However, the pharmaceutical companies (Marketing Authorization Holder) may seek waiver of PBRER and submit the PSUR in earlier format. PBRER is in consistent with latest ICH requirements. The reports are to be submitted quarterly for the first three years following US approval and annually thereafter.

PSUR in United Kingdom: The PSURs are replaced by periodic benefit risk evaluation report (PBRER). The PBRER is a periodic assessment of the risk-benefit balance of a medicinal product. The marketing authorization holder needs to submit the report irrespective of the product is in the market or not. The PBRER provides an analysis of safety, efficacy and effectiveness of the product in the entire life cycle. The report submission periodicity: every six months until the product is placed in the market, every six months for the first two years of introducing the product into the market and annually for the next two years.

Routine PBRERs are not required if the medicinal products fall under the EU's directives. These are: Generics, Products with well established use, Homeopathic medicines and Traditional herbal medicines. PBRERs are jointly assessed by the Medicines and Healthcare Products Regulatory Agency (MHRA) and other European national competent authorities assigned by Pharmacovigilance Risk Assessment Committee (PRAC) or a member country appointed by the Coordination Group for Mutual recognition and Decentralised Procedures. The PRAC issues recommendations for PBRERs for: a centrally authorized product, any mix of centrally authorized products and those under National and EU procedures, and nationally authorised products reflected in the European Union Reference Data (EURD) list. MHRA assesses products for active substances authorized in UK only on an individual basis.

Key Messages

- Submissions of PSURs are post marketing obligations of marketing authorization holders.

- PSURs are systematic review of global safety data which became available to the marketing authorization holders of a marketed medicinal product at pre-defined time interval.

- PSURs are helpful for the marketing authorization holder to ensure the updated product characteristics and patient information leaflets.

- PSURs are valuable Pharmacovigilance data for regulatory authorities to initiate decisions including restricting use or banning a product.

- PSUR begins with approval of the medicinal product and continues for the entire life cycle. The PSURS are to be developed and submitted at predefined time interval as desired by the corresponding regulatory authority.

- Content and format for PSUR are not uniform worldwide. However, ICH guideline E2C (R2) is widely accepted.

- Schedule Y of Drugs and Cosmetics Rule of Drugs and Cosmetics Act (India) specifies the periodicity and format for submission of PSURs.

- Periodic Benefit Risk Evaluation Report has replaced the traditional PSURs in USA and UK and is in consistent of ICH guidelines.

Bibliography

1. 59th Report on the Functioning of the Central Drugs Control Organization, Parliamentary Standing Committee on Health and Family Welfare, 2012.

2. Current Challenges in Pharmacovigilance: Pragmatic Approaches, Reports of CIOMS Working Group V, CIOMS, 2001.

3. Good Pharmacovigilance Practice Guide, Compiled by the Medicines and healthcare Products Regulatory Agency, Pharmaceutical Press, 2010.

4. Guidance for Industry, Providing Postmarket periodic Safety Reports in the ICH E2C (R2) Format, Periodic Benefit-Risk Evaluation Report, Draft Guidance, US Department of Health and Human Services, Food and Drug Administration, Centre for Drug evaluation and Research, Centre for Biologics Evaluation and Research, April 2013, accessed at http://www.fda.gov/downloads/drugs/guidancecomplianceregulatoryinform ation/guidances/ucm346564.pdf on 08 May 2015.

5. Guru Prasad Mohanta, Textbook on Clinical Research: A Guide for Aspiring Professionals and Professionals, PharmaMed Press, 2011.

6. Medicines, medical devices and blood regulation and safety guidance, Periodic benefit risk evaluation reports for medicinal products, 18 December 2014, accessed at https://www.gov.uk/periodic-benefit-risk-evaluation-reports-for-medicinal-products on 8 May 2015.

Chapter 9

Pharmacogenetics in Pharmacovigilance

"The only true wisdom is knowing you know nothing".

Socrates

After reading this chapter, you should be able to understand and appreciate:
• Why different persons respond to medicines differently.
• Influence of genetic variations in medicine action especially causing ADRs.
• Generic markers as risk indicators.
• Classical examples showing genetic basis of ADRs.
• Importance of Pharmacogenetics ensuring safe and more effective medicines.

The inter–individual variability in response to medication is well known. The genetic factors that affect the kinetics and dynamics of medicines play a greater role in determining the individual's risk of non-response or toxicity. Genes affect the way in which the body processes and responds to drugs. Genetic differences explain some of the inter-individual variability in patients' response to some medicines. The variation in gene coding for drug metabolizing enzymes, drug transporters, drug receptors and targets account for a significant portion of the observed heterogeneity in drug response across population. The study of genetically determined variations in drug response is called Pharmacogenetics. In addition to the genetic polymorphism, there are many factors which are responsible for variation in drug response: age of the patient, size – weight and height or body mass index, pregnancy, co-morbidity and renal or liver damage.

Adverse Effects of Codeine

CYP2D6 genotype influences the response to codeine. Poor metabolisers do not convert codeine efficiently to morphine and they get little analgesic effect from codeine. On the other hand, ultra-rapid metabolisers may experience morphine toxicity. High level of morphine can result in breathing difficulty, which may be fatal. 5-10% of Caucasians (human race of Europe, Western Asia, parts of India and North Africa) are poor metabolisers. 29% of North African and Ethiopian populations are ultra-rapid metabolizers and about 6 percent of African American, Caucasian and Greek populations too have similar issues.

Codeine related deaths in children following tonsillectomy have been linked to ultra-rapid metabolism. Children were given codeine for pain relief after surgery that resulted in death of few children [2012]. The adverse drug reporting system of USFDA identified 10 deaths and three over dosage associated with codeine during 1969 to 2012. The USFDA has issued a black box warning for codeine use in children after tonsillectomy.

While it is difficult to know the metabolising status of the individual without genetic testing, it is preferable not to use codeine in children following tonsil removal and to use alternatives for pain management. CYP2D6 genotyping is not routine before prescribing codeine.

The genetically based variations in drug response are primarily caused by mutations of DNA, which result in structural changes of proteins involved in different pharmacokinetic phases of absorption, distribution, metabolism and elimination as well as in drug receptor interactions. Much of the individual's pharmacogenetic response is attributed to the difference in metabolism called genetic polymorphism. The genetic polymorphism is the inter-individual differences in DNA sequences at a specific chromosomal location that exist at a frequency of more than 1% at general population. The two alleles (alternate form of genes) at a given gene locus comprise the genotype. The influence of genotype on phenotype is measurable. The genotype is the genetic code in the cell and the phenotype is the expression and observable traits. Though pharmacognetics have wide application in medical sciences, this chapter restricts the discussion related to Adverse Drug Reactions.

The effect of age on the impact of genetic polymorphism should be considered. The enzyme and transport proteins involved in the pharmacokinetic of a drug may be different in young paediatric patients than in adults as a consequence of different regulation of gene expression. Such differences are mainly expected in new born infants, infants and toddler. There is expression of CYP3A7 in new born and post natal increase in CYP2C9, 2C19 and 3A4 expression in the first year after birth. When a significant impact of a genetic polymorphism on the pharmacokinetics of a drug and/or risk of adverse drug reaction has been established in adults, the potential consequences in the paediatric population should also be considered.

Genetic susceptibility to Adverse Drug Reactions has been established for a number of drugs. Some clinically significant issues are narrated below. Of the CYP enzymes involved in drug metabolism, CYP2C9, CYP2C19 and CYP2D6 are polymorphically expressed clinically important enzymes. The CYP2D6 poor metaboliser phenotype is found in 5-10% of Caucasians and North Americans of African descent and about 1-2% of Asian subjects. The molecular basis for lack of CYP2D6 is explainable. With the present genotyping technologies, CYP2D6 poor metabolisers can be easily identified. The poor metaboliser phenotype for CYP2D6 is reported to cause insufficient metabolism in many therapeutic classes. CYP2C19 (or, mephenytoin hydroxylase) deficiency is found in 3-5% of the Caucasian population and in about 20% of the Asian population.

Warfarin and Genetic Variation

Warfarin reduces blood's ability to clot and prevents blood clots in vein, arteries and heart. It acts by blocking the liver's production of certain clotting factors and has been extensively used in deep venous thrombosis, pulmonary embolus, and in atrial fibrillation. The dose of warfarin needs to be closely monitored and adjusted to achieve appropriate balance between the anti-clotting benefits and serious risk of life threatening bleeding. The two genes are found to influence the effect of warfarin. The gene CYP2C9 is used by the liver cells to make an enzyme that breaks down warfarin. Because of variation in gene type some people metabolise warfarin more slowly than others. Patients with this gene variant (slow metabolisers) require less warfarin to achieve the same anti-clotting effect. With the same normal dose, these patients experience toxicity. The variant of second gene, VKORC1 (Vitamin K epOxide Reductase Complex subunit 1), cause patients to have increased sensitivity to warfarin and requires lower dosing. Vitamin K obtained from diet or vitamin supplements interferes with warfarin. Vitamin K helps the blood clot. Genetic variation in the VKORC1 influences warfarin dosing by three fold than CYP2C9. Realizing the influence of genetic variation in safe warfarin therapy, USFDA (2007) encouraged genetic tests for appropriate dosing. However, recent studies reported in New England

Journal of Medicine (2013) provide strong evidence that genetic testing of warfarin responsiveness does not provide any meaningful benefit to patients being started with warfarin.

Hypersensitivity Syndrome of Abacavir

Abacavir is a nucleoside analogue used in the treatment of AIDS. About 5-9% of the patients develop hypersensitive reactions of which 94% develop the reactions in first 6 weeks of treatment. The hypersensitive reactions are: skin rash, gastrointestinal and respiratory (dyspnea, cough, and pharyngitis) manifestations and re-challenge shock. Failure to recognise these reactions and continued treatment is associated with fatalities. The treatment for these reactions is to stop using abacavir. Re-treatment with abacavir can cause serious allergic reactions including anaphylactic shock.

The study has shown that several genetic markers are associated with abacavir hypersensitivity. But HLA-B*5701 alone serves as an excellent predictive abacavir hypersensitivity syndrome. There is lower risk of hypersensitivity in blacks but it is preferable to screen both black and white population. It is recommended that screening of HLA-B*5701 before starting any abacavir containing regimen on any patient. A positive test indicates that the person is susceptible and the drug should not be given. Though HLA-B*5701 is an excellent tool for detecting abacavir hypersensitivity, the negative test result does not absolutely rule out hypersensitivity. The genetic test is conducted in blood or saliva sample.

Aspirin Adverse Effects

Aspirin has been widely used at low dose to prevent cardiovascular events due to its anti-platelet activity. A new research claims that the common genetic variation in the gene for catechol-O-methyltransferase (COMT) may alter the action of aspirin and harm the persons. COMT is a key enzyme in the metabolism of catecholamines (epinephrine, norepinephrine, and dopamine). These hormones have good influence in hypertension. The study reported that individuals who are homozygous for the enzyme's high-activity valine form, the "val/vals," have been shown to have lower levels of catecholamines compared to individuals who are homozygous for the enzyme's low-activity methionine form, the "met/mets". It is found that the 23% of the women who were 'val/vals' were naturally protected against incident cardiovascular disease.

However, when the women with the val/val polymorphism were allocated aspirin, this natural protection was eliminated. The study showed that val/val women who were randomly assigned aspirin had more cardiovascular events than the val/vals who were assigned placebo; while women, who were met/met, had fewer cardiovascular events when assigned aspirin compared to placebo.

As COMT genetic variant is very common, it may be necessary to individualize the therapy based on genetic profile.

Clopidogrel Adverse Effects

Clopidogrel is used to prevent serious or life threatening problems with the heart and blood vessels in people who had stroke, heart attack, or severe chest pain. It works by preventing platelets from collecting and forming clots that may cause stroke or heart attack. This is a prodrug which is metabolised mainly by CYP2C19 to produce active metabolite that inhibits platelet aggregation. In patients who are CYP2C19 poor metaboliser, less of active metabolite is formed which may result in serious clinical implications: stent thrombosis, myocardial infarction or even death. Based on study reports, the product information of Clopidogrel was updated in European Union to include information related to an increased risk of cardiovascular events with reduced CYP2C19 function due to genetic variant in the gene coding for the CYP2C19 protein. Similar safety concern is also an issue when Clopidogrel is used with CYP2C19 inhibitors like proton pump inhibitors.

Some Clinically significant Adverse Drug Response associated with pharmacogenetics.

Drug	Adverse Response	Responsible Polymorphic Gene
Warfarin (for preventing blood cloting)	Haemorrhage in poor metabolisers	CYP2C9
Irinotecan (for colon or rectal cancer)	Neutropenia	UGT1A1*28
Albuterol (for asthma and COPD)	Asthma control result is based on argino geno type or glycine geno type	β2 Adrenergic receptor
Pravastatin (for cholesterol lowering)	Reduced cholesterol lowering response	CETP

Contd...

Drug	Adverse Response	Responsible Polymorphic Gene
Zileuton (Leukotriene synthesis inhibitor used in asthma)	Variation in response	5-Lipoxygenase
Abacavir (for HIV)	Hypersensitivity	HLA-B*5701
Primaquine (for Malaria)	Haemolytic anaemia (in deficient enzyme patients)	G6PD
Azathioprine (for prevention of treatment rejection and severe rheumatoid arthritis)	Myelosuppression (TPM deficient patients accumulate excessive thioguanine nucleotide)	Thiopurine S-methyltransferase (TPM)
6-mercaptopurine (for acute lymphocytic leukaemia)	Neutropenia and other toxicity	TPMT*2, *3A, *3B, *3C
Gefitnib (for lung cancer)	Diarrhoea	ABCG2Q141K
Isoniazid (for TB)	Hepatotoxic	CYP2E1*1 and NAT2
Tranilast (anti-allergic)	Hyper-bilirubinemia	UGT1A1*28
Allopurinol (for Gout)	Severe Cutaneous	HLA-B*5801
Carbamazepine (for seizure)	Steven Johnson Syndrome (highest risk in persons of Asian Ancestry)	HLA-B*1502

Valuable information can be generated from well documented case reports including information on the relationship between biomarkers (geno type or pheno type) and the clinical features of adverse drug reactions. Spontaneous ADR reports related to possible genetic polymorphism could be the important data source for signal generation or risk evaluation. Well documented case reports may lead to product information change and/or trigger pharmacogenetic research. Description of genomic biomarker information in the product information is essential and the testing the patients may be essential. Medicine induced harm is a public health issue. The pharmacogenomics promise a clearer path to predicting in whom the harm is most likely to occur. Once predicted, it would ensure right medicine to right person thus promoting safety and efficacy. However, the evaluation of economic burden of the ADRs and the cost effectiveness of the pharmacogenetic tests is crucial.

Key Messages

- The variation in gene coding for drug metabolizing enzymes, drug transporters, drug receptors and targets contribute significantly for heterogeneity in drug response across population.

- The genetically based variations in drug response are primarily caused by mutation of DNA which affects pharmacokinetics and drug-receptor interactions. Much of the individual pharmacogenetic response is attributed due to difference in metabolism (genetic polymorphism).

- Genetic susceptibility to adverse drug reactions is established for a number of drugs.

- Spontaneous ADR reports related to genetic polymorphism is an important data source for signal generation or risk evaluation. Pharmacogenetic tests helps in identifying patients in whom the harm is most likely to occur.

Bibliography

1. Guideline on key aspects for use of pharmacogenomic methodologies in the Pharmacovigilance evaluation of medicinal products, Draft, European Medicine Agency, 2014.

2. Roger Walker and Cate Whittlesea, Clinical Pharmacy and Therapeutics, Fifth Edition, Churchil Livingstone, Elsevier, 2012.

3. Ronald D. Mann and Elizabeth B. Andrews (Editors), Pharmacovigilance, Second Edition, John Wiley and Sons, Ltd., 2007.

Chapter 10

Ethical Consideration in Pharmacovigilance

"One must educate the public that seldom does a patient receive the best treatment"

The Flexner Report

After reading this chapter, you should be able to understand and appreciate:
• Whether there is need of observing / complying with ethical requirements for biomedical research.
• Main ethical issues.

Introduction

The medicines are essential for preventing and treating diseases or illnesses. They have harmful effects too. Until the medicines have been in use in diverse population over a long period of time, there are substantial uncertainties on benefit and risks of these medicines. The Pharmacovigilance activities are concerned with detection and documentation of these risks in an attempt to promote safe use of medicines. Regulatory authorities and pharmaceutical companies continue monitoring the drugs while they are in market. The patient and reporter identifiability are important requirements in Pharmacovigilance. They assure the existence of a real person that can be verified or validated in some way. Activities involving human subjects (patients) require ethical consideration.

Main bioethical principles: Ethical principles of biomedical research in human beings are mainly comprised of:

- Non- Maleficence (Do no harm);
- Beneficence (Fruitful result, Do good);
- Autonomy (Respect for persons); and
- Justice (Distributive justice, equitable distribution of risks and benefits).

The potential benefits to the participants, anticipated risks and the compensation thereof, unexpected consequences and the procedures proposed to tackle are covered under first two principles (Non-Maleficence and Beneficence). Informed consent, and privacy and confidentiality of the data are covered under the third point (Autonomy). The principles of justice require that the fruit of research is equitably shared amongst the beneficiaries and research participants. All clinical or biomedical research needs to comply with these requirements. They are the part of Good Clinical Practice guidelines.

Randomized control trials in post marketing phase: Safety monitoring of approved medicines may be broadly divided into two types: Post-Marketing Surveillance (Phase-IV of Clinical Trials, a responsibility of the pharmaceutical company) and routine documentation of adverse drug reaction (Pharmacovigilance programme of Drug Regulatory Authority). Post Marketing Research questions focus on drug's risk and such study designs provide safety evidence of sufficient quality for decision making. When post-marketing randomized control trials are conducted by the pharmaceutical companies, it is essential to protect patients' or participants' rights and interest. Post-Marketing Randomized Control Trials (RCT) are justified in the following conditions:

- A regulatory decision cannot be taken on the basis of available evidence or evidence that could be obtained through observational studies;
- RCTs can be properly designed and implemented to generate evidence for a responsible regulatory decision;
- The regulatory authority will use the trial results in making a regulatory decision in a timely manner; and
- RCT has provision to protect the rights and interest of participants.

Informed consent and confidentiality in PV: The Pharmacovigilance activities are neither clinical trials nor research activities (studies). They are just observational data collection activities without any intervention in the treatment. These activities are recognised as public health activities. As the PV activities are initiated by the Governments (Regulatory Authorities), the informed consent is not required for collection of data for safety monitoring. However, it is essential to maintain the security, privacy and confidentiality of personal data. Personal identifier is an important requirement of PV to avoid duplication and follow up, if required. As patient identifier is recorded, strict conditions are necessary on maintaining data security. Personal identifiable data of both patients and reporter should not be shared with any other parties including pharmaceutical companies or research groups. The published data including reports should not contain any information that could identify the patients.

The persons responsible for PV activities need to be trained in the strict maintenance of security and confidentiality.

Re-challenge: Perhaps the most powerful pieces of evidence to ascertain causality between adverse drug reaction and the suspected drug is the subsequent re-administration of the medicine. This is called re-challenge. It is a matter of debate whether it is appropriate to perform a re-challenge! A decision to re-administer the suspected drug causing adverse drug reaction is dependent on factors like whether the reaction is reversible, whether it is idiosyncratic etc. Careful judgement of the treating clinician is important. Patient informed consent is essential especially if the adverse reaction is serious or medically important. Re-challenge for scientific interest alone is not ethical. Intentional re-challenge should be carried out only when there is likely to be clinical benefit to the patient. This should be done when the treating physician is of the view that the anticipated result is directly relevant to the patient's treatment and well being.

Key Messages

- "Do no harm, Do good, Respect for persons and equitable distribution of risks and benefits" are the fundamental principles of bioethics.

- PV activities involve with minimal risks (almost nil) and hence ethical consideration is less.

- PV programme initiated by regulatory authority is accepted as public health practice not as research. Hence, does not require the necessity of informed consent.

- PMS (observational Studies) conducted by pharmaceutical companies – no clear guidance on the need of informed consent.

Contd...

> - RCTs conducted as Phase – IV of Clinical Trial requires compliance of ethical requirements.
> - Re-challenge for scientific interest is not appropriate but can be done if it offers clinical benefit to the patients.

Bibliography

1. A Practical Handbook on the Pharmacovigilance of Antiretroviral Medicines, World Health Organization, 2009.

2. Contemporary Ethical Issues in Biomedical and Health Research, Indian Council of Medical Research, August 2007.

3. Current Challenges in Pharmacovigilance: Pragmatic Approaches, Report of CIOMS Working Group V, Geneva, 2001.

Chapter 11

Global Scenario in Pharmacovigilance

"Doctors are men who prescribe medicines of which they know little, to cure diseases of which they know less, in human beings of who they know nothing".

Voltaire

After reading this chapter, you should be able to understand and appreciate:
• The Role and Contribution of International Agencies – WHO, ICH and CIOMS;
• The Pharmacovigilance Systems of other Countries – USA, UK and Australia.

The medicines are used throughout the globe and so are the incidences of adverse events. No medicine is safe all the time for all persons. The occurrence of adverse drug reaction varies from one geographical region to the other due to several factors including the formulation of medicines (locally manufactured), customs and diets, and genetic variations. There are Pharmacovigilance programmes throughout the globe but intensity or extent of programme varies based on economic situation. The rich and industrial countries have robust programme and the poor and developing countries may not have that robust but a programme in one or other form. The international agencies like World Health Organization (WHO), International Council on Harmonization (ICH) and Council for International Organizations of Medical Sciences (CIOMS) have been significantly contributing in promoting Pharmacovigilance activities in an attempt to improve patient safety through safe medications.

World Health Organization

World Health Organization, a specialized health agency of United Nations (but not subordinate to UN), started functioning on 7[th]April 1948 with an objective "the attainment by all peoples' of highest level of health". This 7th April, day of adoption of WHO's constitution, is celebrated as World Health Day every year. It has the mandate to develop, establish and promote international standards (on safety, purity and potency) with respect to food, biological and pharmaceutical and similar products.

The thalidomide disaster in 1961 (details can be seen elsewhere in the book) raised international concern on unsafe medications. A Resolution (WHA16.36) of Sixteenth World Health Assembly in 1963 re-affirming the need for early action in regard to rapid dissemination of information on adverse drug reaction led to the creation of the WHO Pilot Research Project for International Drug Monitoring in 1968. The purpose of the project was to develop an internationally acceptable system for detecting previously unknown or poorly understood adverse effects of medicines.

The Pilot Research Project for International Drug Monitoring of 1968 is now grown into a full- fledged WHO programme and is currently coordinated by the Uppsala Monitoring Centre. The Essential Medicines and Health Products (EMP) division of Health Systems and Innovations (HIS) cluster is responsible for the pharmacovigilance activities. WHO programme began just with ten countries contributing to the international database in 1968 and now 120 countries contributing. India joined the WHO programme in 1998. The WHO database is now enriched with more than 10 million case reports which testify the success story of WHO programme. The programme has brought together all the countries with one common vision of preventing patient harm. The 50th Anniversary of WHO Programme for International Drug Monitoring was celebrated on 5-9th November 2018.

---

3 S Tools for Enhancing PV in Low and Middle Income Countries: WHO and Bill & Melinda Gates Foundation have introduced "Smart Safety Surveillance" (or, 3 S) to establish the proof of concept for strategies for building or strengthening the PV System in LMICs. This is a risk based approach for new products that have not been introduced into reference regulatory market but are fast tracked approved. Three products are identified: Bedaquiline (for MDR TB), Tafenoquine (for *Plasmodium vivax*) and Dotutegravir (for HIV during pregnancy).

The WHO Collaborating Centres:

- The Netherlands Pharmacovigilance Centre Lareb as WHO Collaborating Centre for Pharmacovigilance in Education and Patient Reporting. It is trying to develop curriculum and initiated the process of teach the teachers programme for promoting pharmacovigilance education.

- Indian Pharmacopoeia Commission, the National Coordination Centre of National Pharmacovigilance Programme of India, is the WHO Collaborating Centre for Pharmacovigilance in Public Health Programmes and Regulatory Services.

The WHO has published several booklets and documents which are useful in sensitizing and promoting pharmacovigilance activities. The WHO Pharmaceuticals Newsletter and WHO Drug Information are important publications through which WHO disseminate safety information.The WHO programme has developed a standardized adverse reaction terminology (WHO ART) and a comprehensive index of reported drugs (WHO DD). The WHO Drug Dictionary is unique in its coverageof drugs marketed throughout the world.

> **Open Access to Drug Safety Database:** The World Health Organization has recently launched a new open access drug safety database called VigiAccess. VigiAccess is a new web based application that allows everyone to access information on reported cases of adverse events related to over 1,50,000 medicine and vaccines. More than 10 million cases reported from various countries to the WHO database can be accessed now at: www.vigiaccess.org.

Uppsala Monitoring Centre: The UMC is an independent foundation and a centre for international services and scientific research. Its priorities are the safety of the patients and safe and effective use of medicines in every part of the world.

The UMC has been carrying out the WHO's international drug monitoring activities since 1978. It has celebrated 40th Anniversary on 5-9 November 2018 in Geneva along with WHO's 50th Anniversary. As a collaborating centre, it adheres to the WHO policies and works in close association with WHO headquarter. But organizationally and professionally it is distinct from WHO. It focuses on early detection of potential issues relating to use and safety of medicines. The main activities of UMC on pharmacovigilance are:

- Screening and analysing international adverse reaction data;

- Supporting effective communication of the most focused, up-to-date scientific information;

- Providing tools for data entry, management, retrieval, reference and research;

- Alerting regulating authorities of member countries about potential drug safety issues; and

- Capacity building through education and training in setting up and running national pharmacovigilance programmes as well as in using the UMC Tools.

The UMC has developed and uses several software tools to help the participating National Centres in international drug monitoring programme. These include VigiFlow, VigiBase, VigiMine, VigiMed, VigiSearch and VigiLyze.

- ***Vigi flow***: This is a simple web based individual case safety report (ICSR) management system that improves all aspects of ADR reporting. ICSR data can be manually entered into VigiFlow. Once a report is complete and committed the first version of the ICSR is generated and automatically saved in in global database called VigiBase. It is possible to retrieve reports for amendment or follow up.

- ***Vigi base***: This is the WHO's global ICSR database consisting of all reports received from member countries since 1968. This computerized database has information recorded in a structured and hierarchical form to allow for easy and flexible retrieval and analysis of data.

- ***Vigi mine***: It provides access to statistical data on all drug – ADR pairs available in VigiBase. VigiMine allows filtering of the results on a number of statistical criteria and stratification by age, sex, country and year of reporting. It reflects the statistical changes too.

- ***Vigi med***: This is a web based forum for people working in National Centres of WHO programme to have easy access to safety concerns in other countries, to check regulatory status and to expedite the sharing of drug information.

- ***Vigi search***: This is a search tool that provides access to all case reports in VigiBase and searching across multiple drugs and ADRs simultaneously even using a lot of filters. The data can be accessed on an overview level and viewed from number of aspects including individual case report.

- *Vigi lyze*: This is a powerful search and analysis tool that provides access to VigiBase. It can be used to have global, regional or national view of an identified ADR and monitor international patient safety data. It offers international comparison with national spontaneous reporting data and provides access to ADR information of drugs which are not yet available for use in national market. The unique feature of this tool is that the results are instantly available both in tabular and graphic forms.

Each member state collects, processes and evaluates adverse drug reaction reports and submits the information to the WHO database. Case reports submitted on agreed format to the WHO VigiBase are checked for technical correctness and incorporated into the international database. They are screened periodically for new and serious reaction/s. The flow of information from national centres to the WHO database is described graphically.

International Council on Harmonization(ICH): The International Council on Harmonization of Technical Requirements for Pharmaceuticals for Human Use (ICH) provides platform for regulatory authorities and pharmaceutical industries of European Union, USA and Japan to design common guidelines for the development and registration of medicines. Though the guidelines are meant for these three regions but these regions have maximum consumption of medicines. Hence, the other countries are also interested on ICH guidelines as marketing of medicinal products becoming global. India too exports medicines to more than 200 countries including USA, UK, and Japan.

ICH was established in April 1990 and since then it has developed several guidelines, through consultative process, on Quality, Safety, Efficacy and Multidisciplinary. The pharmacovigilance guidelines are developed under safety guidelines. The safety guidelines cover the requirements of pre-clinical testing. The pharmacovigilance guidelines are:

- E2A – Clinical Safety Data Management [Definitions and Standards for Expedited Reporting]
- E2B(R3) – Clinical Safety Data Management [Data Elements for Transmission of Individual Case Safety Reports]

- E2B(R3) – Implementation [Electronic Transmission of Individual Case Safety Reports]
- E2C(R2) – Periodic Benefit : Risk Evaluation Report
- E2D – Post Approval Safety Data Management [Definitions and Standards for Expedited Reporting]
- E2E – Pharmacovigilance Planning
- E2F – Development Safety Update Report

Council for International Organization of Medical Sciences (CIOMS): The CIOMS is an international not for profit organization established by WHO and United Nations Educational, Scientific and Cultural Organization (UNESCO) in 1949. It facilitates and promotes international activities in the field of biomedical sciences. In addition to other areas of works, the CIOMS has initiated activities on 'safety requirements for use of drugs' and 'assessment of and monitoring of adverse drug reactions and pharmacogenetics'. Through its working groups, CIOMS developed recommendations or guidance in the area of international reporting of adverse drug reactions including introduction of standardized reporting form [Copy is enclosed in the Appendix], international reporting of periodic drug safety update reports, core clinical safety information on drugs, evaluation of benefit/risk balance, current challenges of Pharmacovigilance, management of safety information from clinical trials, development safety update reports and signal detection in pharmacovigilance. These guidance documents are very helpful for all stake holders from industry to regulatory agencies.

Many of the recommendations of CIOMS are adopted by ICH. This has contributed significant impact on international drug regulation.

Pharmacovigilance in United Kingdom: Like several other countries the United Kingdom too initiated the systematic way of monitoring of adverse drug reactions soon after the outbreak of thalidomide disaster in 1960s.The Commission on Human Medicines (COHM) of Medicines and Healthcare Products Regulatory Agency (MHRA), an executive agency of Department of Health, is responsible for Pharmacovigilance activities.

The Committee on Safety of Drugs (CSD) of UK headed by Sir Derrick Dunlop had introduced the spontaneous reporting scheme in 1964 asking the members of the medical and dental profession to promptly report the details of any untoward condition in a patient which might be the result of drug treatment. It was known as 'Yellow Card System'. Now too it is known by the same name though pharmacovigilance has no association with yellow colour. The important features of the scheme were:

- Suspected adverse reactions should be reported;
- It was the responsibility of the doctor or dentist to submit report;
- There should not be delay in reporting; and
- Report and reporter's confidentiality was promised.

With the establishment of Licensing Authority in 1971, the Committee on Safety of Drugs was absorbed into it and new Committee was evolved as 'Committee on Safety of Medicines' (CSM). The terminology 'Drug' was thought to be too emotive and hence replaced with 'Medicine'.

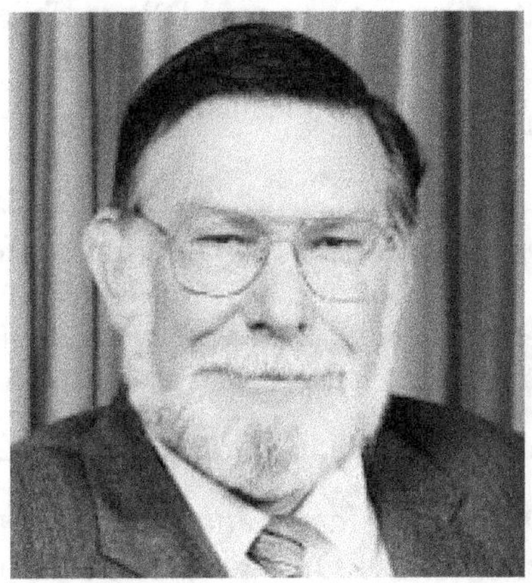

Professor William Inman, a polio affected doctor confined to wheel chair, is credited for developing Yellow Card System in UK for voluntary reporting of Adverse Drug Reaction. His study linking contraceptive pill with thrombosis led to the reduced dose of hormone without reducing the efficacy. This earned him the accolade "Father of the mini pill". He was the first to use the term Post Marketing Surveillance (PMS). Realizing the limitation of spontaneous reporting, he introduced another system for the Prescription Event Monitoring.

There have been several changes in the design of Yellow Card reporting form as the programme expanded. Initially it was the doctors or dentists who were authorized to submit the reports, now it is open to all healthcare professionals including nurses and pharmacists to patients. While for some countries like France, Norway, Sweden, and Spain, reporting of adverse drug reactions are compulsory; in UK it is voluntary. In order to promote reporting, the yellow cards are made available as a part of British National Formulary (BNF) and prescription pads.

The voluntary reporting forms are accepted by MHRA/COHM from both healthcare professionals and members of public. Reports are also received from marketing authorization holders [It is compulsory]. For established products, the MHRA requires that the healthcare professionals report only serious suspected adverse drug reactions. For new products, MHRA encourages the reporting of all suspected adverse reactions. Special attention is given on ADRs in children and elderly and on herbal medicines. Though data is obtained from wide sources, spontaneous reporting system is the main source for pharmacovigilance activities.

Orange Card Reporting: Orange card reporting is a separate initiative of MHRA in collaboration with British Paediatric Surveillance Unit (BPSU) (now known as Royal College of Paediatrics and Child Health) where consultant paediatricians are encouraged to report particular disorders under surveillance in children to the BPSU.

MHRA has ADR online information tracking (ADROIT)database. The reports are entered to ADROIT and MHRA evaluates them to assess the causal relationship between the drugs and reported reactions. Then agency identifies the possible risk factors. The marketing authorization holders have access to ADROIT and there are provisions of exchange of pharmacovigilance data electronically. The MHRA communicates the regulatory decisions through circulation of 'Current Problems in Pharmacovigilance Bulletin' to doctors and pharmacists. In order to disseminate urgent hazard warning "Dear Healthcare Professionals" letters are sent by post and electronically. The fact sheets and safety alerts are placed in website too.

UK was one of the founding members of WHO programme on International Drug Monitoring. Being a member of the European Union, the PV guidance of EU is applicable in UK.

Pharmacovigilance in United States of America

The US FDA is responsible for safety monitoring of medicines and it continues to assess the benefit–risk profile throughout the life cycle of the product. The primary purpose of the pharmacovigilance is the generation of signals or hypothesis of a potential adverse drug effect association. USFDA safety information and adverse event reporting programme is known as MedWatch.

Database: The safety signals may arise from different sources, but the most common is the voluntary or spontaneous case reporting to the regional or National pharmacovigilance centres or FDA. The healthcare professionals or patients voluntarily send the ADR case reports either to manufacturer or to FDA. The report received by FDA either from healthcare professionals, patients or manufacturers are entered into FDA Adverse Event Reporting System (FAERS). *The significant feature is that the database, FAERS, contains not just the ADR reports but also reports on medication errors. The modern pharmacovigilance includes the medication error within its domain.* FAERS is the repository of ADR and medication error.

Report submission: Individual reporter like health professionals (physicians, pharmacists, nurses, and others) or consumers (patients, family members, lawyers and others) can directly submit the adverse event reports to the USFDA. This is voluntary. The manufacturers have the mandatory obligation to submit the reports: A serious ADR is to be submitted within 15 days of the receipt of the report. For most non-prescription products manufacturers are not required to submit the ADR reports to FDA. The format for submitting the report is available in MedWatch website. For the interest of the readers it is kept in appendix. The electronic submission system is also practiced.

Processing of reports: Serious unlabelled ADR reports submitted by manufacturers, Serious ADR reports (labeled or unlabelled) submitted directly to the FDA by healthcare professionals or consumers and reports of selected important medical events are evaluated by clinical reviewers in the Centre for Drug Evaluation and Research (CDER) and the Centre for Biologics Evaluation and Research (CBER). If potential safety concern is identified in FAERS, further evaluation is performed. Then further investigation including computer search of entire database of adverse event reports, literature review, drug usage data and incidence rate are done.

An analysis of the safety issue is then presented to the medical reviewing division responsible for ongoing regulation of the drug. If the signal is strong enough, the regulatory decision such as labeling changes, restricting the use of drug, communicating new safety information to the public and withdrawal from the market is initiated by the FDA.

The MedWatch uses e-mail communication to disseminate new safety information to the healthcare professionals. MedWatch receives reports of serious adverse events for all medical products except vaccines. The vaccine safety monitoring programme is known as "Post Licensure Rapid Immunization Safety Monitoring (PRISM)" Programme.

Pharmacovigilance in Australia: The Office of Medicine Safety Monitoring (OMSM), a branch of Therapeutic Good Administration (TGA) is the responsible authority for safety monitoring of medicines in Australia. TGA is the medicine regulatory authority and is a unit of Australian Government Department of Health and Aging (under Therapeutic Goods Act 1989). TGA has established pharmacovigilance system for the collection and evaluation of information relevant to the benefit to risk balance of registered medicinal products.

Each sponsor or manufacturer of registered medicine must have appropriate pharmacovigilance system in place in order to assure responsibility and liability for its product in the market and to assure that appropriate action can be taken when necessary. The company should have a medically qualified person responsible for pharmacovigilance. The separate sponsor may have same qualified person.

Report submission: The spontaneous adverse event reporting is voluntary in Australia. The healthcare professionals, patients and consumers may report to the sponsors or manufacturers or directly to TGA through Adverse Drug Reaction Advisory Committee (ADRAC) using "Blue Card". The report can be submitted by post to The Secretary, ADRAC, and no postage is necessary if posted in Australia.

ADRAC was formed in 1970 to advise TGA on safety of medicines.

All serious adverse drug reaction reports whether expected or unexpected received by sponsor from healthcare professionals, patients, and consumers are to be reported to ADRAC in an expedited manner [within 15 calendar days]. Cases from worldwide literature review and reports from post-registration studies are also to be reported within 15 days of receipt.

Sponsors are not required to submit the serious reports of foreign origin on an expedited basis. On the other hand, sponsors are required to advise the TGA within 72 hours of any significant safety issue identified as a result of ongoing review process or action taken by foreign regulatory authority. Significant safety issue means withdrawal or suspension of availability of the product; additional information like contraindication added to an approved drug; and modification of alert.

The non-serious ADR reports should be submitted only on request from TGA or included in PSUR.

Web based reporting system is available.

Pharmacovigilance Requirement for Sponsor of
Registered and Listed Medicines

Report Type	Method / Format of Report	Reporting Time Limit
Serious adverse reaction	Blue Card / CIOMS Form / Online Reporting Form	Within 15 calendar days
Significant safety issue	In writing to post-marketing surveillance branch by facsimile or e.mail	Within 72 hours of receipt
Non-serious adverse events	In requested format	As PSUR or as asked by TGA

The sponsor is required to submit PSUR annually for the first three years after the date of approval letter. The first report must be submitted not later than 15 calendar months after approval. The subsequent report must be submitted at least annually from the date of submission of first report.

Processing of reports: TGA's Office of Medicine Safety Monitoring receives reports of suspected adverse events associated with prescription medicines, vaccines, OTC medicines and complementary medicines. On receipt of reports, they are reviewed by professional staff. Reports involving serious reactions or recently marketed drugs are reviewed by adverse drug reaction committee, a sub-committee of Australian Drug Evaluation Committee (ADEC).

After the medical review, if any new safety information is required to be disseminated, the new safety information is circulated to the healthcare professionals through Australian ADRAC bulletin.

Australia participates in International Drug Monitoring Programme managed by Uppsala Centre.

Key Messages

- WHO Programme for International Drug Monitoring was started as a pilot research project in 1968.

- WHO Programme is now coordinated by the Uppsala Monitoring Centre (UMC) in Sweden. The UMC is the WHO collaborating centre for international drug monitoring. 120 countries are currently contributing to the WHO database.

- The Netherlands Pharmacovigilance Centre Lareb is the WHO collaborating centre for pharmacovigilance in education and patient reporting.

- UMC developed several information technology based tools to help the participating national centres: VigiFlow, VigiBase, VigiMine, VigiMed, VigiSearch and VigiLyze.

- CIOMS, an associate of WHO, offers a forum for policy makers, pharmaceutical industries, government agencies and academics to make recommendation on the communication of safety information between regulators and pharmaceutical industries.

- ICH, a platform of drug regulation authorities and pharmaceutical industries of European Union, USA and Japan, has several guidelines on quality, safety and efficacy and multidisciplinary guidance on harmonizing the requirements for registration of medicines for human use. The pharmacovigilance guidelines come under efficacy guidance.

- In UK, the pharmacovigilance activities are managed by Commission on Human Medicine under MHRA. The programme is dependent on voluntary reporting of suspected adverse drug reactions by healthcare professionals and the members of public. The programme is called Yellow Card System. UK was one of the founding members of WHO programme on International Drug Monitoring.

- In USA, FDA is the regulatory authority for safety monitoring of drugs and other medicinal products including medical devices and vaccines. The adverse event monitoring of products other than vaccines are managed through MedWatch. The US programme includes medication error too in pharmacovigilance domain. The adverse events data base is called FAERS. For healthcare professionals and consumers, reporting to FDA is voluntary while for manufacturers it is mandatory.

- Office of Medicine Safety Monitoring of Therapeutic Goods Administration is the agency responsible for pharmacovigilance (safety monitoring) activities in Australia. It is necessary that the sponsor must have appropriate pharmacovigilance system with qualified person being responsible. Spontaneous reporting by the healthcare professionals and patients is voluntary and is managed throughBlue Card System. Sponsor is required to submit serious adverse event reports within 15 calendar days. It is not mandatory to submit the non-serious adverse events in expedited way but as PSUR.

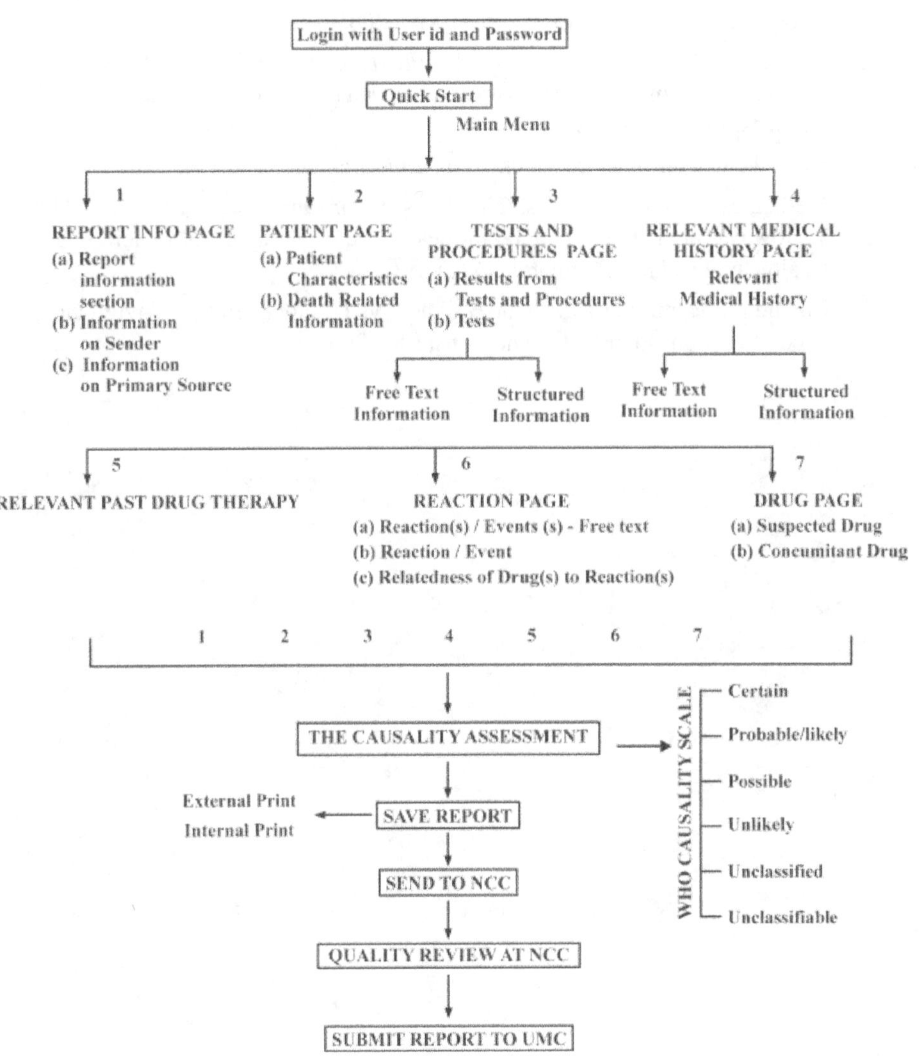

Login with User id and Password
Quick Start
Main Menu
1
REPORT INFO PAGE
(a) Report information section
(b) Information on Sender
(c) Information on Primary Source
2
PATIENT PAGE
(a) Patient Characteristics
(b) Death Related Information
3
TESTS AND PROCEDURES PAGE
(a) Results from Tests and Procedures
(b) Tests
Free Text Information
Structured Information
4
RELEVANT MEDICAL HISTORY PAGE
Relevant Medical History
Free Text Information
Structured Information
5
RELEVANT PAST DRUG THERAPY
6
REACTION PAGE
(a) Reaction(s) / Events (s) - Free text
(b) Reaction / Event
(c) Relatedness of Drug(s) to Reaction(s)
7
DRUG PAGE
(a) Suspected Drug
(b) Concumitant Drug
1 2 3 4 5 6 7
THE CAUSALITY ASSESSMENT
WHO CAUSALITY SCALE
Certain
Probable/likely
Possible
Unlikely
Unclassified
Unclassifiable
External Print
Internal Print
SAVE REPORT
SEND TO NCC
QUALITY REVIEW AT NCC
SUBMIT REPORT TO UMC

Bibliography

1. Australian Guideline for Pharmacovigilance Responsibilities of Sponsors of Registered Medicines Regulated by Drug Safety and Evaluation Branch, Australian Government Department of Health and Aging, Therapeutic Goods Administration, Amended 31 May 2005.

2. Guidance for Industry, Good Pharmacovigilance Practices and Pharmacoepidemiologic Assessment, US Department of Health and Human Services, FDA, March 2005.

3. http://www.who-umc.org accessed on 25 March 2015.

4. Medicines, medical devices, blood regulation and safety guidance, The Yellow Card Scheme: guidance for healthcare professionals, Medicines and Healthcare Products Regulatory Authority, 23 January 2015.

5. Ronald D. Mann and Elizabeth B. Andrews (Editors), Pharmacovigilance, Second Edition, John Wiley and Sons, Ltd., 2007.

Chapter 12

Pharmacovigilance of Ayurveda, Siddha, Unani and Homeopathic Drugs

All substances are poisonous, there is none which is not a poison; the right dose differentiates a poison from a remedy.

Paracelsus

After reading this chapter, you should be able to understand and appreciate:
• The basic philosophies of Ayurveda, Siddha, Unani and Homeopathy (ASU) Medicines.
• The need of Pharmacovigilance of Indian Systems of Medicines and Homeopathy.
• Historical Account of Pharmacovigilance of Indian Systems of Medicine.
• Salient points of National Pharmacovigilance Programmes of ASU&H Medicines.
• Challenges of Safety Surveillance of ASU&H Medicines.

In spite of tremendous developments in the field of modern medicines, the people of India still have limited access to them. A large section of the population continue to rely on the Indian Systems of Medicine (ISM) for their health care for many reasons such as easy availability and affordability. People too believe that they are from natural source and thus are safer compared to modern medicines. Indian Systems of Medicine, a conglomerate of Ayurveda, Siddha and Unani (ASU), has a long history. The popular belief that the medicines of natural origin are harmless and free from side effects is not true. Various studies have shown the serious issues with respect to herbs' safety. The presence of toxic materials in the ASU medicines   are reported in reputed scientific journals. The detection of heavy metals in these products further causes safety concern. The presence of heavy metals in medicinal products at a concentration beyond the acceptable limit can cause serious health hazards including kidney failure. Homeopathy, though not originated in India, has penetrated so well into the roots and tradition of the country that it has been accepted as one of the National System of Medicines. Though usually considered safe when appropriately used, safety issues of the homeopathic medicines can't be ignored especially when unsafe starting materials are used. Hence, the Government of India has launched Pharmacovigilance of ASU &H medicines.

Ayurveda, aptly known as 'Science of Life', is an ancient Indian healthcare system and its history can be traced back to 2500 BC or so. The distinguished feature of Ayurveda is the holistic nature with which it considers a human being in totality and takes into consideration his relationship with the environment. It is known for its comprehensive approach involving life style modulation, biopurification therapy and use of palliative remedies and avoidance of factors that are predisposing or precipitating for disease genesis. Accordingly to Ayurveda, the whole world as well as the human beings are made up of five basic elements *[Earth (Prithvi); Water (Jal); Fire (Agni); Air (Vayu) and Ether (Akasha)]* and are governed by three *doshas* (humours): *Vata, Pitta* and *Kapha*. The balanced state of three *doshas* maintains the body functions and the imbalance causes diseases. Ayurveda aims counteracting the imbalances of three *doshas*. The Ayurvedic medicines are of plant, animal and/or mineral origin and use both single drug or compounded formulations. There are two basic safety issues: inherent presence of toxic substances in the product and unacceptable level of impurities such as microbial contaminants, pesticides, residual solvents and heavy metals. The Drugs and Cosmetics Act of the country has recognized the use of toxic substances in the preparation of Ayurvedic medicines. These substances are listed in Schedule E1 of the Drugs and Cosmetics Rules. During the preparation of medicinal products containing such substances, there is a need to undertake detoxication (called shodhan) as mentioned in authoritative ancient texts. Ayurvedic formulations containing poisonous substances, metals, etc., if not used according to Ayurvedic principles, may show symptoms of toxicity. Ayurvedic experts outline the following factors responsible for toxicity of Ayurvedic medicines:

- *Improper manufacturing process:* The authoritative ancient Ayurvedic texts describe the methods of detoxication of metals used in Ayurveda. When the relevant procedure is not followed but a short cut way is accepted for manufacturing, it can lead to toxicity;

- ***Presence of contaminants:*** The heavy metals are often added deliberately. There is no control over this especially when they are prepared by individuals. One study showed that 17 out of 70 Ayurvedic products tested had heavy metals [Journal of American Medical Association, 2004, 292 (23), 2868-73]. Other studies showed the presence of allopathic drugs like phenytoin and Phenobarbital in Ayurvedic medicines meant for epilepsy treatment and presence of corticosteroids in many Ayurvedic medicines.

- ***Improper use:*** The Ayurvedic medicines are to be used with respect to the vehicle (honey, water etc), relationship with the food (early morning empty stomach, immediately before food, immediately after food, etc.) and dose etc. If the procedure is not adhered to, it may lead to toxicity.

- ***Poor quality:*** Ensuring consistent uniform quality of Ayurvedic medicines is often difficult as the raw materials quality varies widely from source to source and even from the same source at different seasons. The microbial contamination and toxicity of residual solvents used in extraction too cause toxicity to the products.

A married couple showed elevated blood lead levels after taking Ayurvedic herbal medicines, dispensed from an Indian hospital. The male, who had taken the unidentified Ayurvedic medicine for five months was admitted to a hospital in Australia with abdominal pain, nausea and vomiting secondary to lead poisoning. He had a lead level of 120 µg/dL and also high levels of arsenic and mercury. His wife was asymptomatic but also had a high lead level of 40 µg/dL. An acceptable blood concentration for lead is < 10 µg/dL.

The Drugs Regulatory Authority of Australia [Therapeutic Goods Administration (TGA)] has released a statement about the safety of Ayurvedic medicines in Australia, in response to recent research into the toxic content of heavy metals found in some Ayurvedic medicines.

There are several possible explanations for the presence of heavy metals in traditional herbal remedies. Salts of heavy metals (for example those of lead, mercury and arsenic) are used as principal ingredients in some traditional Indian and to a lesser extent in Chinese herbal remedies. In addition, cross-contamination of ingredients can occur between these types of products and products not intended to contain metal salts if manufacturing conditions are not controlled.

Australian Adverse Drug Reaction Bulletin, Vol 26, No. 1, February 2007.

The argument that the Ayurvedic medicines have been in use for thousands of years and there have been very little reports of side effects. This should be the enough evidence of safety of Ayurvedic medicines. The Ayurvedic medicines are no longer prepared or manufactured based on the procedure outlined in the ancient texts but the modern technology. The modernized Ayurvedic medicines cannot be treated on par with the medicines described in ancient authoritative Ayurvedic texts. Safety monitoring of these modern Ayurvedic medicines is a necessity not only in the interest of Ayurveda but also in larger public interest.

Siddha Medicines are of Dravidian origin and is mostly practiced in Tamil Nadu. According to Siddha medicines, there are seven elements: *Saram (plasma), Cheneer (blood), Ooun (muscle), Kozhuppu (fat), Elumbu (bone), Moolai (nerve)*, and *Sukila* or *Inthiriyam (semen)* that are responsible for physical, physiological and psychological functions of the human body. These seven elements are activated by three components or humors:*Vatha (air), Pitha (fire* or *heat* or *energy)* and *Kapha (water)*. It is believed that these humors are in a particular ratio in human body and disturbance of this equilibrium causes illness. Diet, physical activities and environmental conditions are the main cause for disturbance of the humor equilibrium. Most of the Siddha medicines are based on Herbo-minerals and metallic, which are more effective than the single and compound herbal drug preparations. In short, the basic concept of Siddha Medicine is similar to Ayurveda but the mode of preparation is different.

Unani Medicines owe their origin to Greece and the foundation of the system is based on the teaching of Hippocrates, the father modern medicine. Arabs introduced the system to India. The system is based on humoral theory which believes the presence of four humors: *Dam (blood), Balghum (phlegm), Safra (yellow bile)*, and *Sauda (black bile)*. There is unique humoral constitution in every person representing his/her health status. The body has the power of self-preservation or adjustment. The weakening of this power causes imbalance in the humoral composition and causes disease. The medicines help the body to regain this power and restore the humoral balance. The correct diet and digestion are very important to the system. The medicines are mostly of herbal origin though some medicines may be with animal and mineral origin.

Homeopathy owes its genesis to two Greek words: 'Homois' meaning similar and 'Pathos' meaning suffering. It has originated from Europe in the early part of 19th century. Its principle can be described as "Treating diseases with remedies prescribed in minute doses which are capable of producing symptoms similar to the disease when taken by healthy people". This can be simplified as 'Likes are cured by likes'. Homeopathic medicines uses starting materials derived from mineral, herbal and animal origin. There are two potential health hazards associated with homeopathic medicines: related to the raw materials and related to the procedure used to manufacture of finished product. Safety is of particular concern in medicines of biological origin.

Genesis of National pharmacovigilance programme for ayurveda, siddha and unani medicines: On the similar lines of Pharmacovigilance Programme for modern medicines, the National Programme for ASU medicines was initiated with the assistance of World Health Organization Country Office for India in 2008. The Institute for Post Graduate Teaching & Research in Ayurveda, Gujarat Ayurveda University, had taken the lead in developing the protocol for the National Programme. The programme was funded by the Department of AYUSH, Ministry of Health and Family Welfare, Government of India [Now AYUSH is a separate independent Ministry].

The salient points of the programme were:

- The objectives of the programme are classified as: Short term objective – to develop the culture of notification, Medium term objective – to involve healthcare professionals and professional associations in the drug monitoring and information dissemination processes, and Long term objective – to achieve operational efficiencies that would make National Programme a bench mark for global drug monitoring.

- A three tier system was identified: National Pharmacovigilance Resource Centre – One; Regional Pharmacovigilance Centres – Eight; and Peripheral Pharmacovigilance Centres – Thirty. Institute for Post Graduate Teaching & Research in Ayurveda, Gujarat Ayurveda University was appointed as National Pharmacovigilance Resource Centre.

- The programme collected the reports of: all adverse reactions suspected to have caused by the ASU medicines alone or along with any other medicine; all suspected drug interactions; reactions to any other drug which are suspected of significantly affecting patient's management including reactions suspected of causing death, life threatening, hospitalization, disability, congenital anomaly or required intervention to prevent permanent impairment or damage.

- All registered medical practitioners of ASU systems and other paramedical persons involved in healthcare like nurses, pharmacists, primary health care workers etc. were encouraged to report the suspected adverse drug event. The programme did not mandate to accept the report directly from the consumers or patients.

The collected adverse drug reaction data are planned to be handed over confidentially and statistical analysis of the data need to be forwarded to the Department of AYUSH, Government of India.

Following the two safety workshops conducted at Department of Rasasatra of Banaras Hindu University and Gujarat Ayurveda University in late 2007, the WHO Country office for India, impressed the then Department of AYUSH on the need of PV of ASU medicines. The Department consented to initiate the programme with a funding of Rupees Fifty Lakh Rupees. The two officers from the WHO Country Office for India: Dr. DC Katoch (National Consultant and Focal Point for AYUSH Medicines) and Dr. Guru Prasad Mohanta (National Technical Officer for Essential Medicines) conceptualised and provided the technical inputs in developing the protocol for initiating the PV programme which was launched in 2008. Dr. Rabinarayan Acharya, Senior Faculty of Gujarat Ayurveda University shouldered the responsibility of coordinating the first ever PV programme and developing the detail protocols for its operation.

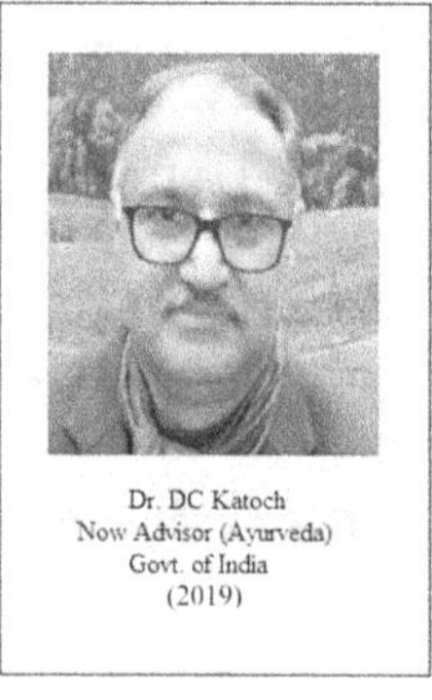

Dr. DC Katoch
Now Advisor (Ayurveda)
Govt. of India
(2019)

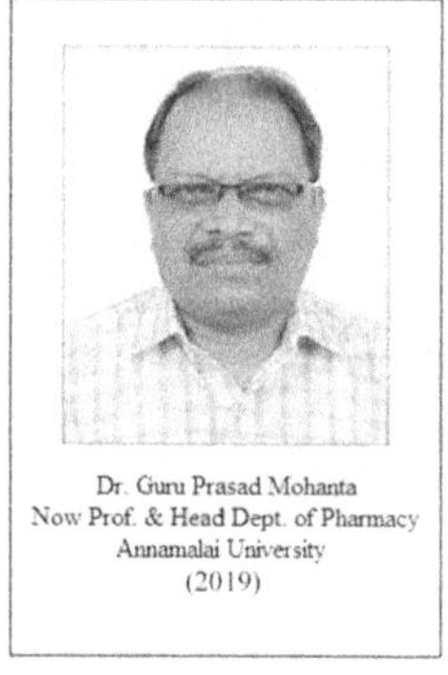

Dr. Guru Prasad Mohanta
Now Prof. & Head Dept. of Pharmacy
Annamalai University
(2019)

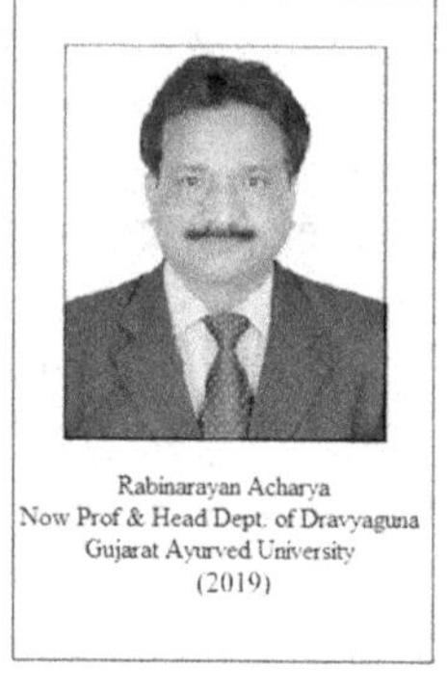

Rabinarayan Acharya
Now Prof & Head Dept. of Dravyaguna
Gujarat Ayurved University
(2019)

National pharmacovigilance programme for ayurveda, siddha, unani and homeopathy drugs: The Ministry of AYUSH, Government of India, has launched a new central scheme in 2017-2018 for promoting Pharmacovigilance of Ayurveda, Siddha, Unani and Homeopathy (ASU&H) medicines. The salient features of the new scheme are:

- Purpose of the Scheme is to:
  - develop the culture of documenting adverse effects and undertake safety monitoring of ASU&H) medicines; and

o conduct surveillance of misleading advertisements appearing in the print and electronic media.

- Structure: It has three tier structure – National Pharmaco-vigilance Centre (NPvCC), Intermediary Pharmacovigilance Centres (IPvCCs) and Peripheral Pharmacovigilance Centres (PPvCCs).

All India Institute of Ayurveda (AIIA), New Delhi, an autonomous institute of Ministry of AYUSH, is the NPvCC. The 5 National Institutes are designated as IPvCCs and 42 AYUSH institutes are recognised as PPvCCs. The All India Institute of Ayurveda is mandated to establish PV network and steer implementation with standard protocol and reporting format, training of coordinators and nodal officers, constitution of various committees and systematic reporting of the progress.

The Central Drug Standard Organization and Indian Pharmacopoeia Commission are associated with the National Programme as Mentor and Guide.

Programme Implementation Committee: The various committees are in place in order to implement the pharmacovigilance programme in a systematic way and is given in the table below:

Committee	Steering & Monitoring Committee	Technical Advisory Committee	Central Signal Detection & Causality Assessment Committee
Members	• Head, DCC, Ministry of AYUSH • Director/ Co-ordinator from NPvCC, AIIA • Coordinator from IPvCC • Representative from CDSCO • Representative from IPC • Representative from PCIM&H	• Chairman of Scientific Body of PCIM&H • Chairmen of APC, UPC, SPC and HPC • Head, DCC, Ministry of AYUSH • Director/Co-ordinator from NPvCC, AIIA • Representative from IPC • Representative from CDSCO • Pharmacology expert from AIIMS/ ICMR • WHO representative of Pharmacovigilance programme (Technical Officer dealing with medicines and pharmacovigilance in WHO country office)	• Coordinator of NPvCC • AYUSH clinical expert • Pharmacy expert of AYUSH system • Pharmacology / Toxicology expert

Administrative Hierarchy of PV of ASU&H Medicines

[Source: https://aiia.gov.in/pharmacovigilance/hierarchy/ accessed on 5th October 2019]

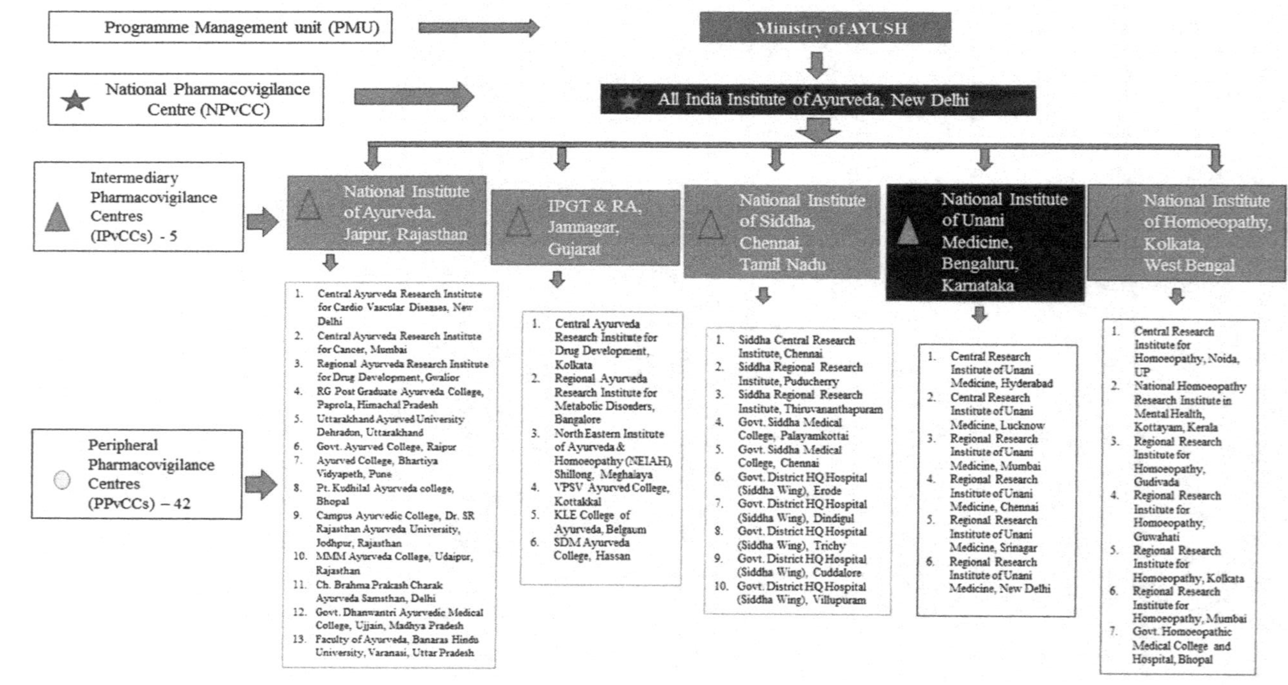

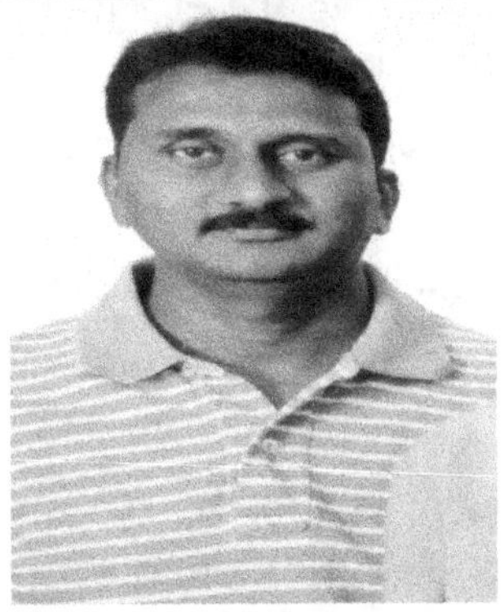

Dr. Galib, Associate Professor of RS and BK, All India Institute of Ayurveda, New Delhi, is the first coordinator and shouldered the responsibility of managing and coordinating the programme. All India Institute of Ayurveda is designated as National Pharmacovigilance Centre for ASU & H Medicines (2019).

Responsibilities of Various Centres:

- **National Pharmacovigilance Coordination Centre:**

  To –

  o Document and monitor the ADRs and misleading advertisements of ASU&H drugs;

  o Seek Periodic Safety Update Reports (PSURs) from ASU&H drug manufacturing companies for all Patent & Proprietary (P&P) drugs;

  o Organise awareness building and capacity building workshops for the stakeholders;

  o Scrutinize the project proposals of the Peripheral Pharmacovigilance Centres in consultation with the concerned Intermediary Centre;

  o Conduct the causality assessment for all the signals regarding the ADRs of ASU&H drugs received from various centres including National Coordination Centre and recommending necessary regulatory action to the Ministry of AYUSH;

- o Provide information to the end users through seminars, drug alerts and other means; and

- o Submit annual proposals and supplementary proposals seeking approval of PAC and PSC.

- **Intermediary Pharmacovigilance Centres (of respective ASU&H system):**

  To –

  - o Document and monitor the ADRS and misleading advertisements of ASU&H drugs;

  - o Collect information regarding the ADRs of ASU&H drugs from the respective Peripheral Pharmacovigilance Centres;

  - o Report the ADRs of ASU&H drugs to the National Pharmacovigilance Centre at regular intervals for causality assessment;

  - o Organise awareness building and capacity building workshops for the stakeholders; and

  - o Scrutinize the project proposals received from Peripheral Centres and forward the same to the National Centre with comments.

- **Peripheral Pharmacovigilance Centres (of respective ASU&H system):**

  To –

  - o Document and monitor the ADRs and misleading advertisements of ASU&H drugs; and

  - o Report the ADRs of ASU&H drugs to the concerned intermediary centre at regular interval.

Monitoring Mechanism: In order to improve the quality and impact of a scheme, it is necessary to use performance monitoring indicators. Performance indicators are measure of project impact, outcomes, outputs and inputs that are monitored during scheme implementation to assess the progress towards scheme objectives. They can also be used to evaluate the scheme's success. The PV of ASU&H scheme has inbuilt monitoring mechanism to measure the efficiency of process, outcomes and impact of the programme. The NPvCC is entrusted with the task of monitoring the programme.

- Process Indicators:
  - o The number of ADR monitoring centres participating in the National PV programme for ASU&H drugs and in the surveillance of advertisements of ASU&H drugs and practices;
  - o Number of personnel trained in ADR monitoring and surveillance of advertisements of ASU&H drugs and practices; and
  - o Funds budgeted for PV programme of ASU&H drugs and funds spent.

- Outcome Indicators:
  - o Number of ADR reports received in a year;
  - o Number of ADR reports processed in a year; and
  - o Number of misleading advertisements of ASU&H drugs and practices reported and processed in a year.

- Impact Indicators:
  - o Number of signals generated and confirmed;
  - o Number of safety related alerts issued by the Ministry of AYUSH; and
  - o Number of misleading advertisements of ASU&H drugs and practices rectified or withdrawn.

Challenges of the PV programme of ASU&H Drugs: While it is anticipated that data generated through the PV programme of ASU&H medicines would provide more confidence among the users and help in promoting global acceptability of Indian System of Medicines; there are many challenges too. More awareness and training programme is to be conducted at various levels to sensitise the ASU&H health professionals on the importance of Pharmacovigilance and benefits of their reporting. Many times, the consumers do take these medicines at their wish considering that they do have no side effects. The consumers even fail or do not think it necessary to tell the physicians about their self-medication. Under such circumstances, it is often difficult to assign the reasons for identified adverse drug reactions. There is no appropriate medicine classification [the anatomical – therapeutic – chemical (ATC)] for all ASU&H medicines and it provides a big challenges coding ASU&H medicines for international comparison.

The WHO has identified the various factors which make the PV of traditional medicines more challenging than the allopathic medicines. All these factors are applicable for ASU&H medicines:

I.   Complex nature of these products:

- Lack of clinical trial data – Systematic clinical trial data is not available and this makes difficult to have safety and efficacy data;

- Chemical Complexity – Most of these products have several hundred of constituents and the effects can't be attributed to one component but a group of related components. As the products composition often varies from manufacturer to manufacturer and sometimes not labelled, it becomes more difficult to identify the suspected drug.

- Non-Uniformity of Products (Non- availability of standards)– The product constituents obtained from plants vary between different batches due to several factors like environment, time of harvest, storage, process and drying. As no single constituent is responsible for effect(s), it is difficult to determine pharmacokinetics, pharmacodynamics, and toxicity;

- Quality Assurance and Quality Control –The quality of raw materials is the critical factor that decides the quality of the product. The source of raw materials, especially from plant origin, often vary widely and so as their quality. The quality varies depending on the geographic region, time of harvest, storage, and manufacturing process. It is not possible to have similar quality control and quality assurance system like what is followed for allopathic medicines;

- Lack of Technical Expertise –Lack of skilled manpower and facilities to identify the drug related issues is a constraint on safety monitoring of traditional medicines; and

- Possible interaction – Though some interaction data are available, for majority of the products data on interaction with allopathic medicines or food is not available.

II. Insufficient information and lack of access to reliable information: There is little information base for these products except the information provided by the manufacturers. The manufactures information may not be unbiased and reliable. This lack of unbiased information makes the work of pharmacovigilance professionals difficult. Misleading advertisements, often unregulated, causes challenges in documenting the use of products. Hence, the PV of ASU&H medicines has mandate for surveillance of misleading advertisements with false claims.

III. Botanical Nomenclature: The nomenclature of plants is not consistent. Plants are main source for ASU&H medicines. This leads to confusion in the documentation process.

IV. Non-existence of safety monitoring system: The healthcare providers are not trained on safety monitoring of Indian Systems of Medicine. Besides, the traditional belief that the system uses the medicines which are prepared from natural resources and hence safe. This leads to either under reporting or no report. The under reporting is true even

Global resurgence of Ayurveda especially its herbal component necessitates the need of its scientific validation in terms of safety and efficacy. The National PV Programme of ASU&H drugs has to go a long way establishing the scientific evidence of safety of ISM. Now, with AYUSH as a separate ministry, it is expected that the programme would receive greater attention in public interest as well as in popularising ISM globally.

In addition to the quality and safety concerns of ASU&H medicines, the improper drug information in the form of advertisement is also an issue. The misleading advertisements cause serious harm on public health as these medicines are often used by the patients themselves without doctor's advice. About 809 complaints of advertisements pertaining to Ayush and herbal medicines/products have been received by the Ministry during the period from April, 2015 to March, 2018. Advertising Standards Council of India (ASCI) reported 732 complaints in the period from 20th January, 2017 to 19th January, 2018. The Government added the surveillance of misleading advertisement to the pharmacovigilance programme. In brief, the Pharmacovigilance Programme of ASU&H medicines aims to facilitate detection of potentially unsafe ASU&H medicines and misleading advertisements; and providing evidence to the government to take regulatory decisions against them.

Key Messages

- Ayurvedic (Vedic origin), Siddha (Dravidian origin), Unani (Greek origin) and Homeopathy (German origin) have long history of use in India. They are either herbal or herbo-mineral products.

- The popular believe that herbs or natural means safe is not true. There are two basic safety issues: inherent presence of toxic substances in the product and unacceptable level of microbial counts, pesticides, residual solvents and heavy metals.

- The safety issues of ASU medicines are reported in many scientific publications.

- The National Pharmacovigilance Programme for ASU medicines was initiated during 2008 with Institute for Post Graduate Teaching & Research in Ayurveda, Gujarat Ayurveda University, as National Resource Centre. Later the Ministry of AYUSH has launched a Central Scheme 'Pharmacovigilance of ASU&H Medicines' during 2017-2018.

- The Central Scheme differ from earlier programme in few significant way: Budgetary provision is made, Homeopathic medicines are brought under the PV programme, Surveillance of Misleading Advertisement is made part of PV programme and Central Institutes are exclusively included as Centres. It has inbuilt evaluation indicators: process indicators, outcome indicators and impact indicators.

- There are several constraints in promoting pharmacovigilance activities of ASU&H medicines. These include: Complexity of these medicines, non-existence of appropriate classification system (ATC), insufficient reliable and unbiased information, Confusing botanical nomenclature, virtual non-existence of safety monitoring system, ignorance of consumers and ASU&H professionals on safety issues, product variation from manufacturer to manufacturer and lack of appropriate classification of medicines.

Bibliography

1. Ayurveda and its Scientific Aspects: Opportunities for Globalization, Department of AYUSH and Council of Scientific and Industrial Research, Government of India, 2006.

2. Galib and Rabinarayan Acharya, National PPharmacovigilance Programme for Ayurveda, Siddha and Unani Drugs, AYU, 29 (4), 2008.

3. Guidelines for the Regulation of Herbal Medicines in South East Asia Region, WHO – SEARO, 2004.

4. https://aiia.gov.in/pharmacovigilance/ accessed on 2nd October 2019.

5. National Pharmacovigilance Protocol for Ayurveda, Siddha and Unani (ASU) Drugs, National Pharmacovigilance Resource Centre, Gujarat Ayurveda University, 2008.

6. Pharmacovigilance for traditional medicinal products: Why and how, World Health Organization, SEARO, 2017.

7. Safety Issues in the Preparation of Homeopathic Medicines, World Health Organization, 2009.

8. Syed Zia-ur Rahman, Rahat Ali Khan and Abdul Latif, Pharmacovigilance in Unani Medicine – A Challenge, The Pharma Review, July – August, 2011.

9. WHO guidelines on safety monitoring of herbal medicines in pharmacovigilance systems, World Health Organization, Geneva, 2004.

Chapter 13

Materiovigilance in India

"Ultimately, by far the greatest benefit to patient safety will be achieved by increasing the skills and the knowledge of many rather than penalising the very few"

Don Berwick

After reading this chapter, you should be able to understand and appreciate:
• The need and genesis of Materiovigilance programme in India.
• The salient features of National Materiovigilance Programme.
• The organogram and functioning of Materiovigilance Programme of India.
• What are to be reported and what are not to be reported as Medical Device Adverse events?
• Classification of severity of Medical Device Adverse Events.
• The story of one of the biggest medical device disaster which affected India.
• Medical Device Monitoring Programme in US.

Under Indian Regulation (Drugs and Cosmetics Act and the Rules), the medical devices used to be notified as drugs for bringing them under the regulatory control. Realising that the medical devices are different from drugs and they deserve to have separate regulation, the Medical Devices Rules 2017 was notified. The medical devices were brought under the Medical Devices Rules with effect from 2018. Like drugs, the medical devices carry certain degree of risk. The ASR Hip replacement (Artificial Hip Joint) has reported to have caused toxicity to more than 4000 patients in India due to leached metal toxicity. The GOI has fixed the minimum amount of compensation for ASR victims at Rupees 20 Lakh. See the text box for more details.

Realizing the need of adverse events monitoring the Government of India launched Materiovigilance Programme [MvPI] in 2015 in an effort to ensure safety of medical devices. Like Pharmacovigilance Programme of India, this nationwide programme called, Materiovigilance Programme of India (MvPI), is coordinated by the Indian Pharmacopeia Commission. The programme intends to monitor medical device associated adverse events (MDAE), create awareness among health professionals about the importance of MDAE reporting and to monitor the benefit–risk profile of medical devices. It is also meant to generate independent evidence based recommendations on the safety of medical devices and to communicate the findings to all stakeholders. The biotechnology wing of the Sree Chitra Thirunal Institute of Medical Sciences and Technology in Thiruvananthapuram is designated as the national collaborating centre for the programme. There are exclusive 17 MvPI centres in the country. Healthcare Technology Division of National Health System Resource Centre (NHSRC), established under National Health Mission (NHM), provides the technical support.

Objectives of MvPI

The Materiovigilance Programme is launched with the following objectives:

- To establish a nationwide system for vigilance on medical device related adverse events;
- To detect and record suspected serious adverse events associated with medical devices: death / serious deterioration in health status, serious injuries and disability;
- To identify and analyse new signal from the reported cases via active / passive surveillance;
- To perform analysis: Benefit : Risk, Risk Analysis and Causality Analysis;
- To generate evidence based information on medical device and alert the regulators and health care professionals;
- To support regulatory authorities in the decision making process;
- To communicate safety information to all stake holders with an aim to minimise the risk;
- To create awareness among healthcare professionals about the significance of MDAE reporting;

- To emerge as National Centre of Excellence;
- To collaborate with other National Centres for exchange of information and data management; and
- To provide consultancy and training support to other National Materiovigilance Centres.

Short Term Goals	Long Term goals

- To develop and implement Materio-vigilance System in India.
- To enroll initially 10 Medical Colleges in the Programme covering North, South, East and West of India.
- To encourage clinicians, biomedical engineers / clinical engineers, hospital technology managers, pharmacists, nurses, technicians, medical device manufacturers for reporting Adverse Events related to medical devices.
- To compile adverse events reports, analyse, and submit medical reports to medical device regulators.
- To *suo motu* analyse and prepare reports on medical adverse events.
- To promote voluntary registration of medical device manufacturers to:
  - Report adverse events to IPC-NCC.
  - Undertake root cause analysis for deterioration or failure on any of their medical device and report to IPC – NCC.
  - Report corrective or preventive action taken in regards to potential adverse events / near miss incidents / adverse events / recalls related to medical devices.
	- To expand the Materiovigilance Programme to all hospitals (Government and Private) and Centres of public health programmes located across India.
	- To develop and implement electronic reporting system (e-reporting).
	- To provide feedbacks and submit progress or status report to all individuals reporting adverse events using MvPI MDAE form.
	- To issue medical device alert to general public or healthcare profession via e-mail or text message.
	- To monitor correcting action taken by the manufacturers in response to report submitted by Materiovigilance Programme Centre.
	- To support health system to procure medical devices which are safe for use.
	- To make Materiovigilance reporting mandatory for medical device manufacturers or their authorised representative for marketing or sale of medical advices in India.
	- To make adverse event reporting of medical device mandatory for all healthcare providers under Clinical Establishment Act.

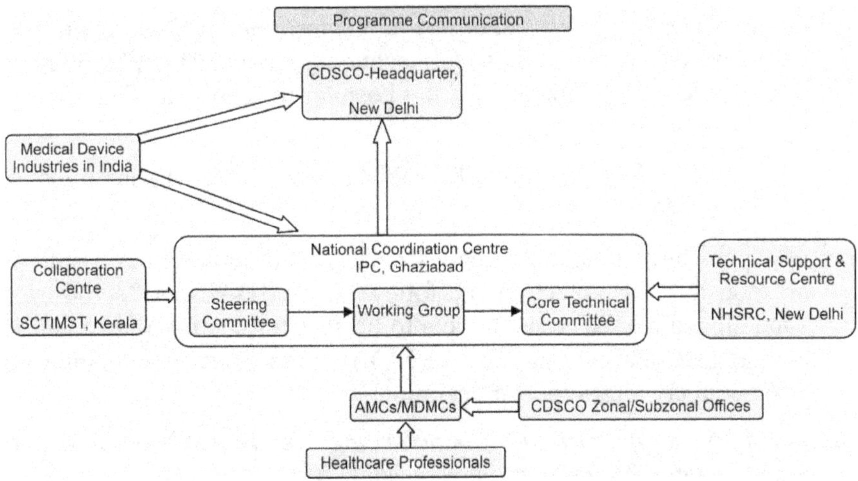

[Source: Materiovigilance Programme of India, Guidance Document, Version 1.1]

Responsibilities of Stakeholders

The MvPI has the following stakeholders: Medical Device Monitoring Centres (MDMC), National Collaborating Centre (SCTIMST), National Coordination Centre (NCC), Central Drugs Standard Control Organization (CDSCO) and National Health System Resource Centre (NHSRC). The responsibilities of the stakeholders are given below:

Responsibilities of Medical Device Monitoring Centre: Each MDMC has a coordinator and a research associate.

- *Responsibilities of the coordinator:* The coordinator is responsible for-

    o Proper functioning of the concerned MDMC with everyone adhering SOPs;

    o Checking completeness of a valid case, failure mode effect analysis, causality assessment and scrutinizing the MDAE reports as per SOPs. He/she should call meeting in MDMC after initial analysis for further deliberation with experts;

    o Sending the consolidated monthly reports of its MDMC to its NCC;

    o Proactively investigate and gather risk based information as and when reported by global regulators. The information should be reported to NCC;

- o Sensitizing / Encouraging clinicians, biomedical engineers, clinical engineers, hospital technology managers, pharmacists, nurses, and technicians of the hospital to report Medical Device Adverse Events; and

- o Sending feedback to all healthcare professionals involved in reporting.

- **Responsibilities of research associate:** The research associate is responsible for collection and follow up of MDAEs. All scrutinized and signed MDAE reports have to be sent for central assessment in National Collaborating Centre. MDAE report has to be submitted immediately after report preparation.

***Responsibilities of National Collaborating Centre* (SCTIMST):** The National Collaborating Centre is responsible for:

- Receiving and collating all adverse events reported from MDMC;

- Coordinating with respective MDMC for further follow up / analysis in case of a serious adverse event;

- Data collection, collation, analysis, signal detection, base line study and communication of its outcome to NCC;

- Organising continuous professional development education programme on Materiovigilance at various zones;

- Conducting periodic training and workshops for all enrolled MDMCs; and

- Database maintenance.

***Responsibilities of National Coordination Centre* (NCC):** The NCC is responsible for –

- Coordinating with all partners of MvPI and organizing steering committee & working group meeting;

- Recognition of new medical device adverse event monitoring centres of public and private hospitals across the country;

- Recruitment of manpower and appointing MvPI staff working under the administrative control of NCC;

- Sending the directly received reports from SCTIMST to the nearest MDMC for processing;

- Analyse data received from SCTIMST and recommend CDSCO for regulatory action;

- Publication and dissemination of SOPs, guidance documents, Newsletter, training manuals etc. with support from NHSRC and SCTIMST;

- Providing financial support to SCTIMST and NHSRC for procurement of technical Documents; and

- Providing assistance to NHSRC for organizing MvPI awareness programme among medical device manufacturers / health care organizations.

Responsibilities of Central Drugs Standard Control Organization (CDSCO): The CSDSCO is the National Drugs Regulatory Authority. It is responsible for –

- Taking appropriate regulatory decision and actions on the basis of recommendation of NCC;

- Joining International Medical Device Regulators' Forum (IMDRF) and Asian Harmonization Working Party (AHWP) and other forums organized by regulatory authorities of other countries for exchange of post-market safety information globally via National Competent Authority Report (NCAR) form exchange programme;

- Organizing meeting with NCC, SCTIMST & NHSRC for continuing monitoring of medical device safety; and

- Auditing / inspecting MDMCs and National Collaborating Centre with NCC officials providing administrative support to run MvPI.

Responsibilities of National Health System Resource Centre (NHSRC): The NHSRC is responsible for –

- Providing technical support / guidance for the preparations of SOPs, guidance documents, newsletters, training manuals etc.;

- Providing support in identification of new MDMC and intimating the same to NCC;

- Providing Technical Support for National Collaborating Centre and National Coordination Centre activities including training;

- Drafting terms of reference for various positions under MvPI. It is to explore possibility of integrating data mining / data analytics to adverse event reports;

- Providing technical advice on setting up of online system for adverse events data collection and release of medical device alerts via e. mail / sms; and

- Promoting adverse events monitoring activities among medical device manufacturers / health care organization.

Reporting of Medical Device Adverse Events*:* The manufacturers and healthcare service providers can report adverse events associated with medical devices. The reporting form, Medical Device Adverse Event Reporting Form (MDAERF), is given in Appendix.

Reporting by Medical Devices Manufacturers: The manufacturers should voluntarily report the incident event to National Coordination Centre. The following types of adverse events are to be reported:

- A malfunction or deterioration in the characteristics or performance of the medical device;
- An incorrect or out of specification test result;
- An inaccuracy in labelling, instructions for use and promotional materials. Inaccurate includes omissions and deficiencies;
- Discovery of a serious public health threat. This may include an event that is of significant and unexpected nature and is a potential public health hazard like HIV;
- Increase in user error or application error;
- Recall or field correction notice from other countries; and
- Other information like complaint trend gathered from literatures.

The initial report of an event in MDAE reporting form with remedial action to prevent an unreasonable risk of substantial harm to public health; and events resulting in death or serious public health threat; should be reported within 5 working days of becoming aware of the event.

MDAE or incident in MDAE reporting form with causality assessment report and future preventive or correctives that would be taken in a defined time frame is to be submitted within 30 calendar days.

Reporting by Healthcare Service Providers: They should report to the research associate at Medical Device Monitoring Centre (MDMC). The following types of adverse events are to be reported:

- A malfunction or deterioration in the characteristics or performance of the medical device;
- An incorrect or out of specification test result;
- An inaccuracy in labelling, instructions for use and promotional materials. Inaccurate includes omissions and deficiencies;

- Discovery of a serious public health threat. This may include an event that is of significant and unexpected nature and is a potential public health hazard like HIV;
- Increase in user error or application error;
- Information available from other countries; and
- Other information like complaint trend gathered from literatures.

The adverse event or incident in MDAE report form with causality analysis should be submitted within 5 working days of becoming aware of its occurrence. The adverse events with analysis of its root causeshould be submitted within 30 calendar days.

What is NOT to be Reported: The following categories incidents or events need not be reported:

1. When the cause of adverse event is the use of medical device after its recommended shelf life – Example: patient admitted to the hospital with hypoglycaemia due to inappropriate insulin dosage following blood glucose testing result. Investigation showed that the test strip used beyond the expiry date.

2. When deficiency of medical device found by the user prior to its use – However, the user should inform the manufacturer of any deficiency identified prior to the use of a medical device. Example: the packaging is found to be damaged but has the label "Do not use if the package is damaged or opened".

3. When the event is caused by the patient's condition (When the MDMC or manufacturer has the information that the root cause of the event is the patient condition) – MDMC or manufacturer should consult expert (related to clinical discipline and medical device) in making the decision. Example: The patient died after dialysis but had an end stage renal disease. The death was attributed to renal failure.

4. When in built protection mechanism functions correctly and prevented the occurrence of harm – The design features of the medical device protected against causing a hazard. Example: An infusion pump stops due to a malfunction but gives appropriate alarm which is in compliance with the standard and there is no injury.

5. When an expected and foreseeable side effect is associated with the use of medical device – The following causes qualify for this criterion:

   a. Clearly identified in the product labelling;

b. Known clinical events – as found in the clinical trial;

c. Documented in the device master record; and

d. Clinically acceptable patient safety concern.

Example: Patient suffered from claustrophobia (severe anxiety) in the confined space of a MRI machine leading to an injury. MRI has known potential risk of claustrophobia.

6. When the risk of death or serious deterioration of state of health is negligible – when the risk is quantified and found to be negligibly small. Example: The manufacturer has identified a software bug after the release of pacemaker for use. The risk (probability of occurrence of a serious deterioration of state of health) with a particular setting is negligible. The patient experienced no adverse health effects.

Severity of Medical Device Adverse Events: The severity of adverse events associated with use of medical devices are grouped into three categories:

1. Death of patient / user or other person;

2. Serious injury to patient or user or other person – while defining 'serious injury' is difficult, it may be of either life threatening illness or injury, permanent impairment of a body function, cause congenital abnormality or permanent damage to a body structure;

3. No death / serious injury but event might lead to death or serious injury of a patient / user / other person.

The Story of Faulty ASR Hip System:

The DePuy International Limited, a subsidiary of Johnson & Johnson, marketed the Articular Surface Replacement (ASR), a 'metal on metal (MoM)' hip as an alternative to metal head with a polyethylene cup. Metal cup was thought to be more durable than the plastic cup. It was used as hip replacement. Cobalt, Chromium, and Molybdenum are the major constituents of MoM hip implant. There are two types of DePuy's ASR system: ASR XL Acetabular Hip System and Depuy ASR Hip Surfacing System. Of these two, ASR Hip Resurfacing System was only approved for use outside USA and was not available for use in USA. USFDA did not approve this implant because resurfacing was then a new procedure.

Contd...

Globally these systems were introduced in July 2003 and in India in June 2004. First, ASRs were recalled by the company in December 2009 in Australia. In August 2010, there was voluntary recall globally. The reasons for recall was cited as high rate of revision of surgery. The patients fitted with ASRs had undergone tremendous sufferings including vision impairment, tinnitus and heart palpitations. All these adverse effects are perhaps due to metal (cobalt, chromium) toxicity. The ASRs were reported to be faulty. The voluntary recall from India was made in August 2010. The company surrendered the registration and import licence only on April 2012.

The expert committee appointed by the central government to look into the issue of faulty hip joints found that the company has been evasive in providing the information regarding the designs of ASRs, patient details who have been fitted with ASRs, compensation details, follow up of Adverse Drug reaction reports etc. The company appears to be delayed in passing information and awareness about the failure of ASR hip joints. The lapse on this part had definitely increased sufferings and had it been timely, it would have minimised the risks. Sufferings of the ASR fitted patients were described as "Patients had to live a restricted life style with a compromised physical state. They are under pain and agony throughout their life which will also have bearing on their dependents in addition to loss of work." Even after the recall of ASRs in Australia in 2009, DePuy applied for import licence in India in January 2010 which was granted. When recalled in Australia, the company did not alert either the regulatory authorities or the patients immediately. It allowed the ASRs to be fitted into the patients.

Recall alert was issued by CDSCO only on December 2013. This was the time when the company was negotiating with compensation settlement in Australia and USA. The Indian Government woke up only in 2017 to form an expert committee to look into the problems, recall and impact on the patients. The recommendations of the committee were accepted by the Government with partial modification and urged the state governments to frame the state level committee to track the patients. The minimum compensation amount for the affected patient was recommended by the expert committee is Rs 20 lakh and exact amount would be decided by another expert committee based on disability. The Johnson and Johnson agreed for a settlement to around 8000 claimants of USA at USD 2.47 billion and in Australia it was about USD 250 million plus interest and legal cost. The amount of compensation proposed in India is not commensurate

[Extracted from: Guru Prasad Mohanta, Kirtimaya Mishra and PK Manna, *Too late and too less for ASR Hip Joint used Indian victims! Chronicle Pharmabiz, Vol. 18 (51), page 10, November 21, 2018*]

> **Medical Device Reporting (MDR) in USA:** In USA, the MDR regulation requires mandatory reporting by the manufacturers, importers, and device user facilities on certain device related adverse events and product problems to the regulatory agency, FDA. Manufacturers need to report when any of their devices has caused or contributed death or serious injury. Malfunctioning and likely to cause or contribute death or serious injury are also required to be reported.
>
> Importers are required to report to the FDA and the manufacturer when they learn that one of their devices may have caused or contributed to a death or serious injury. The importer must report only to the manufacturer if their imported devices have malfunctioned and would be likely to cause or contribute to a death or serious injury if the malfunction were to recur.
>
> The device user facility like hospital, ambulatory surgical facility, nursing home, outpatient diagnostic facility, or outpatient treatment facility must report a suspected medical device-related death to both the FDA and the manufacturer. User facilities must report a medical device-related serious injury to the manufacturer, or to the FDA if the medical device manufacturer is unknown.A user facility is not required to report a device malfunction, but can voluntarily advise the FDA of such product problems using the voluntary MedWatch Form.
>
> There is Voluntary Malfunction Summary Reporting (VMSR) program which was established in 2018. It permits manufacturers to report certain device malfunction medical device reports (MDRs) in summary form on a quarterly basis. It specifies which malfunctioning are not eligible for VMSR.
>
> **Voluntary Reporting System:** The healthcare professionals, patients, caregivers and consumers to submit voluntary reports of significant adverse events or product problems with medical products to MedWatch, the FDA's Safety Information and Adverse Event Reporting Program. The problems experienced should also be reported.

The medical devices offer opportunities for improved diagnosis and management of diseases. But they carry substantial risk too. This is evident from the withdrawal of faulty ASR orthopaedic implants, recalling of bioresorbable stents by Abbott, reporting of failure of pelvic mesh implants. Even after the introduction into the market for use, their surveillance for continuing on going assessment of safety and efficacy is necessary. Even the most rigorous clinical testing will not be able to answer all safety and effectiveness concerns. The new Medical Device Rule has provision of waiving clinical trials in Indian population, if medical device is approved by the regulatory authorities of US, UK, Australia etc. and marketed for at least two years. This provision is planned to be used to remove regulatory bottlenecks while ensuring the availability and increased access to the state of art devices in the market. This further makes Indian population more vulnerable and need of strengthening Materiovigilance in the country. This is necessary for creation of safer environment in healthcare and a condition for the prevention of adverse events.

Key Messages

- Materiovigilance Programme of India, a Nationwide Programme, was launched in 2015, to monitor adverse events associated with the use of medical devices in an attempt to create a safer environment in healthcare and a condition for the prevention of adverse events.

- Indian Pharmacopeia Commission is the National Coordination Centre; and Biotechnology wing of Sree Chitra Thirunal Institute of Medical Sciences & Technology is the National Collaborating Centre. Health Technology Division of National Health System Resource Centre provides the Technical Support to MvPI.

- In addition to the medical device manufacturers / importers / traders, the staff of clinical establishments: clinicians, biomedical engineers, clinical engineers, hospital technology managers, pharmacists, nurses and technicians can report medical devices events,

- Following events are to be reported: A malfunction or deterioration in the characteristics or performance of the medical device; An incorrect or out of specification test result; An inaccuracy in labelling, instructions for use and promotional materials; Discovery of a serious public health threat; Increase in user error or application error; Recall or field correction notice from other countries; and Other information like complaint trend gathered from literatures.

- Following events need not be reported: When the cause of adverse event is the use of medical device after its recommended shelf life; When deficiency of medical device found by the user prior to its use; When the event is caused by the patient's condition; When in built protection mechanism functions correctly and prevented the occurrence of harm; When an expected and foreseeable side effect is associated with the use of medical device; and When the risk of death or serious deterioration of state of health is negligible.

- The severity of medical device adverse events are classified into three categories: Death of patient / user or other person; Serious injury to patient or user or other person; and No death / serious injury but event might lead to death or serious injury of a patient / user / other person.

- Medical Device Adverse Effect monitoring exists in other countries too. In US, The reports are to be submitted using Medwatch form to USFDA.

Bibliography

1. Guru Prasad Mohanta, Kirtimaya Mishra and PK Manna, *Too late and too less for ASR Hip Joint used Indian victims! Chronicle Pharmabiz, Vol. 18 (51), page 10, November 21, 2018.*

2. https://www.fda.gov/medical-devices/medical-device-safety/medical-device-reporting-mdr-how-report-medical-device-problems Accessed on 24th August 2019.

3. Materiovigilance Programme of India, Guidance Document, Version 1.1.

Chapter 14

Haemovigilance in India

"Experience is making mistakes and learning from them"

Bill Ackman

After reading this chapter, you should be able to understand and appreciate:
• The need and genesis of Haemovigilance Programme.
• The salient features of National Haemovigilance Programme of India.
• The functioning of Haemovigilance Programme of India.
• The classification, causality and types of adverse events that may occur at recipient point of blood or blood product transfusion.
• The responsibilities of staff at blood donation point and blood transfusion point.
• The Haemovigilance system in other countries.

Blood transfusion is a clinical necessity for saving lives and promoting health. Providing safe and adequate blood to the needy should be the responsibility of any health system. The blood for transfusion is obtained from the following types donors: voluntary unpaid, family / replacement, and paid. The World Health Organization (WHO) recommends the mandatory screening of bloods for HIV, Hepatitis B, Hepatitis C, Malaria and Syphilis. However, there are risks of adverse events associated with donation of blood and its components; and with transfusion of blood and blood products to the patients. WHO recommends the establishment of system like 'Haemovigilance' to monitor adverse events at blood donation points as well as at transfusion point. Initially, Haemovigilance was restricted for monitoring adverse events at transfusion practices but later expanded to include adverse events in blood donors to improve donors' safety as well. Haemovigilance is defined as "a set of surveillance procedure covering the whole transfusion chain from collection of blood and its components up to the follow up its components intended to collect and assess information on adverse effects resulting from the use blood products and to prevent their occurrence or reoccurrence".

The term 'Haemovigilance' is derived from the Greek word 'Haema' meaning blood and Latin word 'Vigil' meaning watchful &was coined in France in 1991 in an analogy to the existing term 'Pharmacovigilance'. The Haemovigilance Programme was first launched in France in 1994. India has launched its programme called 'Haemovigilance Programme of India (HvPI)' on 10th December 2012 for assuring patient safety and promote public health. National Institute of Biologicals (NIB) is designated as coordinating centre to collate and analyse data with respect to adverse reactions/ events associated with blood transfusion and blood products administration.

Objectives: The HvPI was launched with the following objectives – To

- Monitor transfusion reactions;
- Create awareness among health care professionals;
- Generate evidence based recommendations;
- Advice CDSCO, the Central Drugs Control Authority, for safety related regulatory decisions;
- Communicate findings to all key stakeholders; and
- Create National and International linkages.

Later, National Blood Donor Vigilance Programme (NBDVP) was initiated with the following objectives:

- To improve donors' safety and satisfactions through monitoring, analysing and researching adverse events;
- To analyse risk factors, implement and evaluate preventive measures;
- To provide evidence based support for improving blood donation process; and
- To reduce the frequency of adverse events and increase donation frequency.

Governance and Functioning: There are two committees appointed under the programme to oversee the governance and functioning of the whole HvPI:

I. A core group: to coordinate the activities of haemovigilance between the medical colleges (haemovigilance centres) and National Coordinating Centre (NIB).

II. An advisory committee:

  a. To finalise the Transfusion Reaction Reporting Form (TRRF);

  b. To provide expert opinion for collection, collation, analysis of haemovigilance data and development of software;

  c. To monitor the functioning and quality of data collected by Adverse Transfusion Reaction Reporting Centres;

  d. To develop training modules and guidelines for implementation of haemovigilance programme under PvPI; and

  e. To develop a road map for linking HvP under PvPI with International Haemovigilance Network.

Flow of Information:

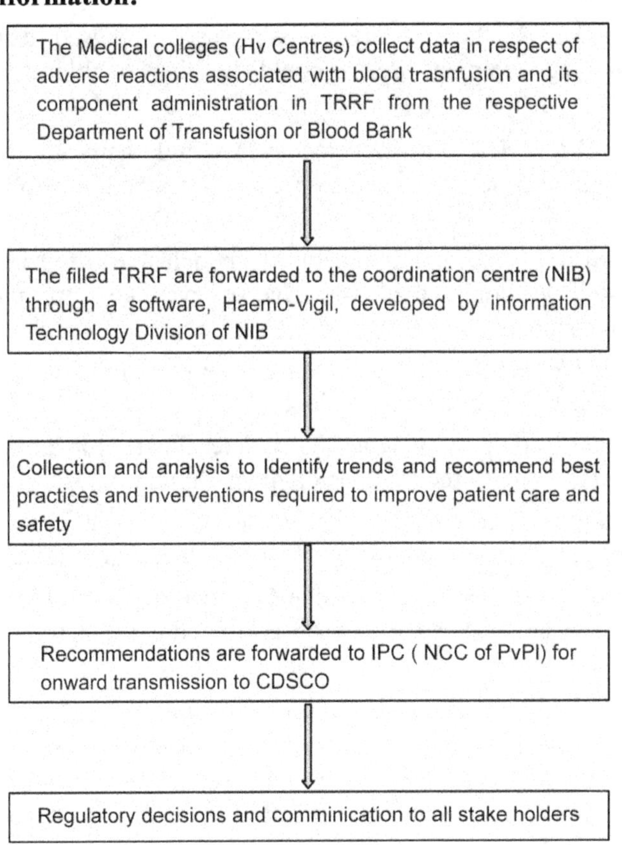

Classification of Adverse Events (Recipient Vigilance): The adverse events following blood or blood product transfusion can be described based on a grading system according to their severity and attributability:

Grade 1 (Non-Severe): The appeared adverse event may require medical intervention such assymptomatic treatment but lack of treatment would not causepermanent damage or impairement of a body function.

Grade 2 (Severe): The appeared adverse event required in patient hospitalization or prolongation of hospitalization directly attributable to the event and / or adverse event resulted in persistent or significant disability or incapacity; or the adverse event necessiated medical or surgical intervention to preclude permanent damage or impairement of a body function.

Grade 3 (Life threatening): the appeared adverse event required a major intervention such as vasopressor, intubation, transfer to intensive care to prevent death.

Garge 4 (Death): the appeared adverse event caused death. In all likelyhood, the recipient death could be due to blood component transfused.

Causality Categories: The adverse events and their association with blood and blood products transfusion can be grouped into following five categories:

    I.   *Definite (Certain)*: If there is conclusive evidence beyond reasonable doubt that the adverse event is attributed to the transfusion;

    II.   *Probable (Likely)*: If the evidence is clearly in favour of attributing adverse event to the transfusion;

    III.   *Possible*: If the evidence is indeterminate for attributing the adverse event to the transfusion or an alternate cause;

    IV.   *Unlikely (Doubtful)*: If the evidence is clearly in favour of attributing the adverse event to causes other than transfusion; and

    V.   *Excluded*: If there is conclusive evidence beyond reasonable doubt that the adverse event can be attributedto the causes other than transfusion.

Classification of Blood Transfusion Reactions: The adverse events following transfusion of blood and blood products can be classified broadly into two categories: Infections and Non-infectious reactions. Infections include the recipient is infected with any of these: HIV, Hepatitis B, Hepatitis C or Malaria.

The Non-Infectious reactions may be acute or delayed. Examples of Acute Non-Infectious Reactions: Acute haemolytic transfusion reaction, febrile non-haemolytic transfusion reaction, transfusion associated acute lung injury, hypotensive reactions, hypokalaemia. Examples of delayed non-infectious reactions: Delayed haemolytic transfusion reaction, delayed serological transfusion reaction, post transfusion purpura, transfusion associated graft versus host disease, haemosiderosis.

Roles and Responsibilities: The World Health Organization has identified the following responsibilities for blood donation centres and transfusion centres:

Haemovigilance in the donation and provision of blood and blood products	Haemovigilance in clinical transfusion
In a national haemovigilance system, blood centres and transfusion services have the following roles and responsibilities: • Donor haemovigilance, including recognition and clinical management of adverse events associated with donation, and their monitoring, reporting, investigation and analysis; • Implementation of policies, guidelines, protocols and standard operating procedures for all processes in the donation and provision of blood and blood products; • Epidemiological surveillance of donors, post-donation information and look-back; • Identification, recording and reporting of: — Near misses, errors and deviations associated with these processes; — Abnormalities in intermediate and finished blood products. • Traceability of each donation from the donor to blood processing, the blood product, its issue to a health-care facility and transfusion to the patient, and vice versa; • Response to notification of a patient adverse event, by retrieval of all blood components associated with the index blood component(s);	In a national haemovigilance system, hospitals and other health-care facilities have the following roles and responsibilities: • Patient haemovigilance, through recognition and clinical management of adverse events associated with transfusion, and their monitoring, reporting, investigation and analysis; • Correct identification of patients, samples and blood products, and appropriate labelling; • Implementation of hospital standards, clinical guidelines and protocols for safe blood transfusion, investigation of adverse events and reporting by clinical services; • Traceability and documentation of transfused blood products in patient records; • Response to product recall and look-back notification; • Active participation in a hospital transfusion committee; • Integration of haemovigilance in the hospital quality system, and mechanisms for taking corrective and preventive actions and monitoring outcomes;

Contd...

• Implementation of haemovigilance as part of the quality system, and mechanisms for taking corrective and preventive actions and monitoring their outcomes; • Training and assessment of staff involved in all steps of the donation and provision of blood and blood products; • Liaison with hospitals: administration, blood banks, transfusion committees and clinical services.	• Training and assessment of staff involved in all steps of clinical transfusion, including clinical decision-making, pre-transfusion sampling, laboratory practice, handling of blood units in the clinical area, bedside administration of transfusion and patient monitoring; • Regular audit of clinical transfusion practices; • Mechanisms for coordination between hospital departments and clinical services, and liaison with blood transfusion services.

Haemovigilance in other Countries: The Haemovigilance programme was first initiated in France in 1994. The United Kingdom was the first country to introduce voluntary reporting system in 1996. Canada, Ireland, the Netherlands, and Denmark have voluntary reporting requirement and their programme is linked to International Haemovigilance Network (IHN).

The Haemovigilance System of different countries have different governance system: Regulatory Authorities are responsible for the programmes of France, Germany, and Switzerland; Blood manufacturers are responsible for programmes of Japan, Singapore and South Africa; and the Medical Societies are responsible for programmes of the Netherlands and United Kingdom.

The WHO website confirms that currently 34 % of hospitals in the African region, 81% in the Americas, 64% in the Eastern Mediterranean, 86% in Europe, 80% in South East Asia and 38% in the Western Pacific have systems for reporting adverse transfusion events. 46% of countries have a Haemovigilance system. The European region has the highest percentage of countries with Haemovigilance systems (76%), followed by the Eastern Mediterranean (53%), the Western Pacific (48%), Africa (38%), South-East Asia (36%), and the Americas (21%).

The Indian Haemovigilance Programme has expanded to include the adverse event monitoring at blood donation point and achieved the status of being a member of International Haemovigilance Network. Enrolling all medical colleges and blood banks under HvPI would further strengthen India's programme and promote public health.

Key Messages

- Haemovigilance is defined as "a set of surveillance procedure covering the whole transfusion chain from collection of blood and its components up to the follow up its components intended to collect and assess information on adverse effects resulting from the use blood products and to prevent their occurrence or reoccurrence".

- Haemovigilance Programme of India is an integral part of Pharmacovigilance Programme of India and the National Institute of Biologicals is the National Coordinating Centre.

- The programme includes the adverse events monitoring during blood and blood products transfusion practices; and adverse events occurring at blood donors' point (NBDVP).

- The adverse events following transfusion of blood and blood products are graded into four categories: Grade 1 (Non-severe), Grade 2 (Severe), Grade 3 (Life threatening) and Grade 4 (Death).

- Based on causality, adverse events at recipient point are classified into: Definite (Certain), Probable (Likely), Possible, Unlikely (Doubtful) and Excluded.

- The blood transfusion reactions are classified into two broad groups: Infections and Non-infectious Reactions.

- WHO has been recommending establishment of Haemovigilance System in all countries. Many countries have already such system but their governance varies among the countries: Regulatory Authorities (France, Germany, and Switzerland); Blood manufacturers (Japan, Singapore and South Africa); and the Medical Societies (the Netherlands and United Kingdom).

Bibliography

1. A guide to establishing national haemovigilance system, World Health Organization, 2016.

2. Bisht A, Marwaha N, Kaur R, Gupta D, Singh S. Haemovigilance Programme of India: Analysis of transfusion reactions reported from January 2013 to April 2016 and key recommendations for blood safety.Asian J Transfus Sci , 12: 1-7, 2018

3. Bisht A, Singh S, Marwaha N, Hemovigilance Program – India, Asian J Transfus Sci, 7, 73-74, 2013.

4. Global Consultation on Haemovigilance 20-22 November 2012, World Health Organization, 2013.

5. Singh *et al*, Review on Haemovigilance Practice in India, World Journal of Pharmacy and Pharmaceutical Sciences, 4(12), 2015.

Chapter 15

Pharmacovigilance of Vaccines

"An old error is always more popular than a new truth"

German Proverb

> **After reading this chapter, you should be able to understand and appreciate:**
>
> - The need of Safety Monitoring of Vaccines;
> - The difference between Safety Monitoring of Vaccines and Medicinal Products;
> - Classification of Adverse Effects Following Immunization;
> - Protocol for Monitoring Adverse Effects Following Immunization;
> - Causality Analysis of AEFI; and
> - Issues of Vaccine Hesitancy.

Vaccines and vaccinations are one of the best medical interventions in medical sciences for promoting public health. Ever since the success of small pox vaccine eradicating the dreaded smallpox from the world, the immunization programmes strengthened worldwide including India to prevent preventable diseases. The Government of India in December 2014 launched 'Mission Indradhanush' to achieve complete immunization for all children by 2020 against seven diseases: diphtheria, whooping cough, tetanus, polio, TB, measles and hepatitis B.

The vaccines are different from other medicinal products. The other medicinal products are meant for patients while the vaccines are basically meant for healthy persons mostly children. Realizing the safety concern of vaccines, the Indian regulation keeps the vaccines as new drugs while all other medicinal products (drugs) are treated as new drugs only for four years of their introduction to market or entry into pharmacopoeia whichever is earlier. The death of even one child during immunization practice not only causes grave psychological issues in the mind of vaccinator, it also threatens the very foundation of basis of immunization. The community loses trust.

The safety monitoring of vaccines is essential like that of other medicinal products. The vaccine pharmacovigilance is defined as the science and activities relating to detection, assessment, understanding, prevention and communication of adverse events following immunization or any other vaccine or immunization related issues. The India's programme is known as 'Adverse Event Following Immunization (AEFI)' Surveillance and Response. The safety of vaccines or AEFI Surveillance system was initiated in 1986 and is monitored by the Division of Adverse Events Following Immunization (AEFI), Ministry of Health and Family Welfare. The goals of AEFI Surveillance are to: minimize the negative impact of AEFI on public health, monitor the quality of vaccine used for immunization, ensure and monitor the quality of immunization services, and reduce morbidity and mortality due to AEFIs.

AEFI is a medical incident that takes place after an immunization causes concern and is believed to have caused by immunization. The details of AEFI are available in Government of India's AEFI Surveillance and Response-Operational Guidelines. The responsibility of reporting depends on the site of vaccination: It is Auxiliary Nurse Midwife (ANM) and medical officers in rural areas; and health workers and medical officers in urban areas. The private practitioners both in rural and urban areas who administer vaccines need to report to the District Health Authority. There are two channels of reporting: Monthly Routine Reporting and immediate serious AEFI reporting. All serious AEFI are to be immediately notified by the first person who identifies the event. The first person should notify the case to the nearest Government Primary Health Centre, Community Health Centre, and /or District Immunization Officer by quickest means of communication.

With collaboration of AEFI Surveillance and Pharmacovigilance Programme of India (PvPI), a reporter can report AEFI cases either to Adverse Drug Reaction Monitoring Centre (AMC) or National Coordinating Centre (NCC). This is an additional method of reporting. The AEFI cases reported to PvPI are further coordinated with National level AEFI Committee and State Expanded Programme Immunization Officers for reporting and investigation.

Difference between Safety Monitoring of Vaccines and Safety Monitoring of Medicinal Products:

1. Vaccines are given to healthy persons and medicinal products are given to sick persons;

2. The vaccines are accepted voluntarily while medicines are taken by the patients without having a choice;

3. Vaccines are usually administered not only for the benefits of the individuals but also for the entire community. Medicine use just benefits the individual;

4. Reporting pathways for AEFIs and Adverse Events of medicinal products is different; and

5. Implication of an adverse event is also different. The entire cohort of the population is affected by the AEFIs while the adverse event of medicinal product affects only a small number of patients.

AEFIs are more important to the health of the population, and of greater interest and more challenging as well. The communication of AEFIs is very critical as misconceptions about vaccine can completely destroy the most cost effective public health programme, immunization.

Classification of AEFI: The reported adverse events can either be true adverse events or coincidental events that are not due to vaccine or immunization process but are temporarily associated with immunization. The AEFI are classified into the following categories:

- **Vaccine Reactions:** The vaccine reactions are further divided into two categories based on cause; and seriousness and frequency:

    I. **Cause Specific Vaccine Reactions**

        o *Vaccine Product Related Reactions:* They are reactions inherent to the vaccine properties and occur even if the vaccine is prepared, handled and administered properly. Most often the exact mechanism of such reactions is poorly understood. Examples: Anaphylactic reactions; Vaccine associated poliomyelitis following oral polio vaccine which contains attenuated live virus.

        o *Vaccine Quality (Defect) Related Reactions:* The reactions are caused or precipitated by a vaccine that is due to one or more quality defects of the vaccine product, including its administration device as provided by the manufacturer. Examples: Insufficient inactivation of wild-type vaccine agent (e.g. wild polio virus) during the manufacturing process; contamination introduced during the manufacturing process. [In 1955, the administration of inactivated polio vaccine caused polio disaster. The polio vaccine used was manufactured by Cutter Laboratories in USA and the investigation showed the presence of live polio virus in the vaccine.]

II. Vaccine Reactions by Seriousness and Frequency

The vaccine reactions may be classified into: 'common, minor reactions'; and 'severe and serious reactions'. Most vaccine reactions are mild and settle on their own. More severe and serious reactions are very rare and generally do not cause long term problems.

a. ***Common, Minor Vaccine Reactions:*** Local reactions, fever, and systemic symptoms can result as a part of the immune response. The vaccine components like aluminium adjuvant, stabilisers or preservatives may too cause reactions. Local reactions like pain, swelling and / or redness at the injection site are expected in about 10% of the vaccines. The following table gives a view of occurrence of adverse events associated with vaccines used under Universal Immunization Programme in India.

Name of the Vaccine	Local Adverse Events (Pain, Swelling and Redness)	Fever (more than 38 °C)	Irritability, Malaise and Systemic Symptoms
BCG	90-95%	-	-
OPV	None	Less than 1%	Less than 1%
Hepatitis B	Adult – up to 15% Children – up to 5 %	1-6 %	-
Hib	5-15 %	2-10 %	-
Pertussis (D_wPT) [D_w = Diphtheria whole cell]	Up to 50 %	Up to 50 %	Up to 55 %
Tetanus	~ 10 %	~ 10 %	~ 25 %
Measles / MR / MMR	~ 10 %	~ 5-15 %	5 % (Rash)
JE live Attenuated	< 1 %	-	-

Source: Immunization Handbook for Medical Officers, Department of Health and Family Welfare, Government of India, 2008.

b. Serious and Severe Vaccine Reactions: An AEFI is considered serious if it results in death, requires hospitalization, results in persistent or significant disability/ incapacity on a cluster (two or more cases) of AEFIs occur in a geographical area. Serious and severe are not same and not interchangeable. Severe is used to describe the intensity of an event (mild, moderate, severe) and serious indicates the life threatening situation. AEFIs that are not minor but not serious too are termed as severe. Example of severe AEFIs: Fever which may be graded as mild or moderate. The example of serious AEFIs: Anaphylaxis.

The rare vaccine reactions are given the table below:

Name of the Vaccine	Reaction	Onset Interval
BCG	Suppurative lymphadenitis	2-6 months
	BCG osteitis	1-12 months
	Disseminated BCG infection	1-12 months
OPV	VAPP†	4-30 days
Hepatitis B	Anaphylaxis	0-1hour
Hib	None	------------
Pertussis (D$_w$PT) [D$_w$ = Diphtheria whole cell] / Pentavalent Vaccine	Persistent (>3 hours) inconsolable screaming	0-24 hour
	Seizures††	0-3 days
	Hypotonic, hypo responsive Episode (HHE)	0-48 our
	Anaphylaxis	0-1 hour
	Encephalopathy§	0-2 days
Tetanus	Brachial neuritis	2-28 days
	Anaphylaxis	0-1 hour
Measles / MR / MMR	Febrile seizures	6-12 days
	Thrombocytopenia	15-35 days
	Anaphylaxis	0-1 hour
	Encephalopathy	6-12 days
Rotavirus	Intussusception	-3-14 days

Source: Immunization Handbook for Medical Officers, Department of Health and Family Welfare, Government of India, 2008.

- **Immunization Error – Related Reactions:** AEFI can occur as a result of inappropriate handling, prescribing or administration of a vaccine. These errors are preventable and hence, it is essential to identify them as this would help taking measures to avoid them. Examples of these immunization are:

a. ***Handling Error in Vaccine / Diluent***: Examples – Exposure to excess heat or cold to vaccine / diluent due to not following cold chain through distribution process. Systemic or local reaction may occur because of changes in physical form of the vaccine. Using vaccines after expiry date may not give protection against the disease because of loss of potency. Use of reconstituted vaccine after the recommended period may lead to contamination usually with *Staphylococcus aureus* which may cause local tenderness and tissue infiltration, vomiting, diarrhoea, cyanosis, high temperature within few hours of administration.

b. ***Prescribing Error / Non-adherence to Recommendation:*** Examples – Failure to adhere to the recommendation on contraindication can cause anaphylaxis, disseminated infection with live attenuated vaccine. Failure to adhere to dose or schedule may cause Systemic and/or local reactions, neurological, muscular, vascular or bony injury due to incorrect injection site, equipment or technique.

c. ***Administration Error:*** Examples – Incorrect sterile technique or inappropriate procedure with a multi-dose vial can cause infection at the site.

- **Immunization Anxiety – Related Reactions:** They are common among the children of above 5 years due to fear or pain of injection rather than the vaccine. These are unrelated to the content of vaccine. Examples are: fainting, light headedness, dizziness, tingling around the mouth. The young children may have vomiting and breathe holding. The anxiety related reactions are more observed in mass immunization programme.

- **Coincidental Events:** The event happens after immunization but are not causally related. A coincidental event is falsely considered to be the reason for immunization. Coincidental adverse events may be preventable.

The vaccines are normally administered in early part of life when infections and other illnesses are common including manifestation of an underlying congenital or neurological condition. In 2010, six infants died within 48 hours of administration of pentavalent vaccine in a country. The vaccination with this was temporarily suspended. The high level investigation showed that three death were coincidental. Of the remaining three, one was due to anaphylaxis and the remaining death reason was inconclusive.

Causality Assessment of AEFI: The causality assessment of reported AEFI is one of the critical components of adverse events surveillance system. Investigations to find out the causal relationship between AEFI and vaccine is important not only to allay public concern over reported adverse events often in lay press but also for taking regulatory decision to remove the vaccine from market. Causality assessment usually does not prove or disprove an association between an event and the immunization; it just assists in determining the level of certainty of such an association.

Causality assessment helps in identification of vaccine related problems; identification of immunization error related problems; excluding coincidental events; detection of potential signals for follow up testing of hypotheses and research; and validation of pre-licensure safety data with comparison with PMS safety data. The quality of causality assessment is dependent on three factors: the performance of AEFI system in terms of responsiveness and effectiveness; availability of appropriate investigation data; and the causality review process.

The causality assessments are performed at different levels: population level, individual level and at signal detection level. There are four pre-requisites for initiating causality analysis: completion of AEFI investigation; availability of complete case details; availability of valid diagnosis for the unfavourable or unintended sign, abnormal laboratory findings, symptom or disease in question; and vaccines administered are known.

The following four steps are involved in causality assessment:

1. Step 1: To determine if AEFI case satisfies minimum criteria for causality assessment;

2. Step 2: To systematically review the relevant and available information to address possible causal aspects of AEFI. The detail check list is given in Appendices.

3. Step 3: Algorithm: Reproduced with permission from WHO's Causality assessment of an adverse event following immunization (AEFI): user manual for the revised WHO classification (Second edition), 2018.

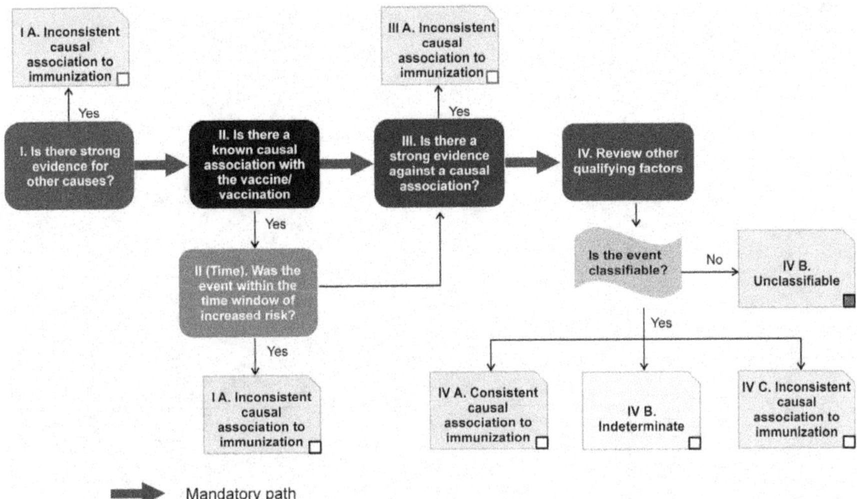

4. Step 4: Classification – To categorise the AEFI's association to the vaccine or vaccination on the basis of the trends determined in the algorithm. The WHO's causality assessment protocol classifies AEFI reports into the four broad categories given in the table:

Category	Type	Sub-Types
A	Consistent causal association to immunization	A1 – related to vaccine product; A2 – vaccine quality defect; A3 – immunization error; and A4 – immunization anxiety
B	Indeterminate	B1 – consistent temporal relationship but insufficient evidence for vaccine causality; and B2 – conflicting evidence or inconsistency about a causal association to immunization
C	Coincidental or inconsistent causal association with immunization	--------
D	Unclassifiable	--------------------

Responsibilities of Stake Holders: The AEFI Organizational Structure of India is given in the diagram given below (reproduced from Guidance for Industry on Pharmacovigilance Requirements for Biological Products, Central Drugs Standard Control Organization, 2017)

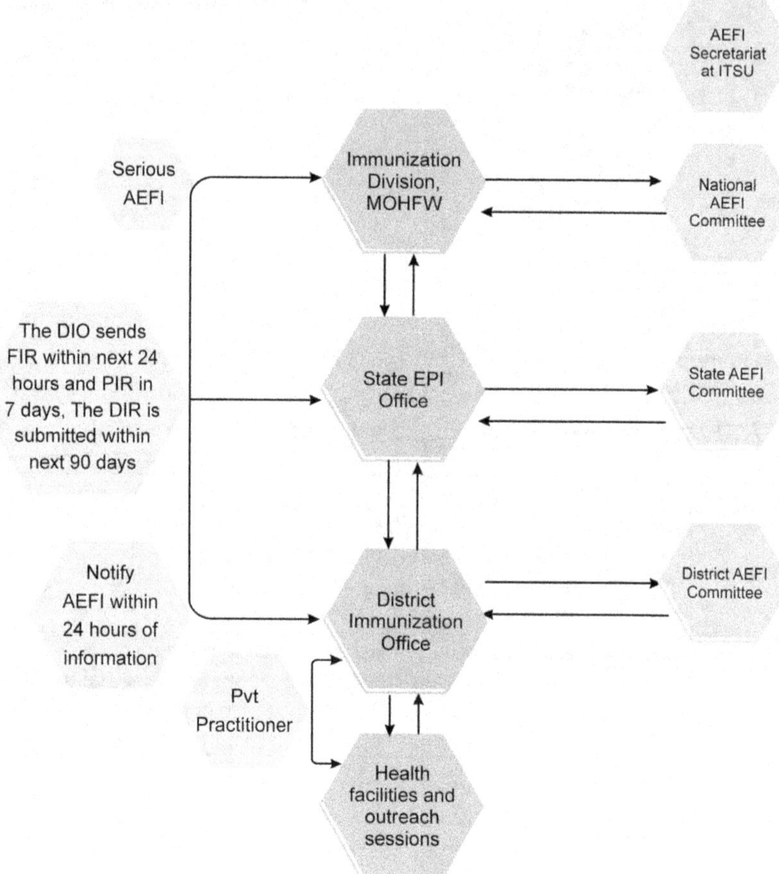

[Reproduced from AEFI, Surveillance and Response, Operational Guidelines, Government of India, 2015]

The responsibilities of various stake holders: authorities, service providers and marketing authorization holders of vaccines are:

a. Responsibilities of Authorities:

Roles and Responsibilities of Authorities in Ensuring Vaccine Safety [http://www.pvpi.in/ne.html#menu3 accessed on 26th October 2019)		
National Coordination Centre (IPC - PvPI)	Adverse Event Following Immunization (AFI) Secretariat	Central Drugs Standard Control Organization (CDSCO)
1. Indian Pharmacopoeia Commission (IPC) functions as National Coordination Centre to monitor, report, collate, and analyse adverse events due to medicines and vaccines.	1. The National AEFI Secretariat, established in Immunization Technical Support Unit (ITSU), is mandated to provide technical support to the National AEFI Surveillance Programme. The Programme is a part of Universal Immunization Programme.	1. This is the National Regulatory Authority empowered to ensure the safety, efficacy, and quality standards of pharmaceutical, medical devices and vaccines.
2. IPC gives recognition to public and private hospitals as adverse drug event monitoring centres (AMC).	2. The Secretariat shares the reported AEFIs with CDSCO on a weekly basis through soft and printed copies.	2. The AEFI Division of the CDSCO functions in close association with PvPI, Immunization & AEFI Cell for continue monitoring of vaccine safety.
3. PvPI team at AMC is responsible for monitoring AEFIs in private and public hospitals of their region. The AMC shall share reported serious AEFIs with District Immunization Officer (DIO) and State Expanded Programme on Immunization Officers immediately.	3. The Secretariat forwards all the AIFI reports received from NCC-PvPI to the concerned zonal consultant for further follow up at the State and District Levels by the SEPIO / DIO to ensure reporting through CRF and investigation PCIF / FCIF.	3. It initiates the regulatory decision based on causality assessment report.

Contd...

4. A serious Individual Case Safety Report (ICSR), due to vaccine, received at NCC should be immediately communicated to AEFI Secretariat and AEFI Division in CDSCO for further action. Non-serious ICSRs need to be communicated on monthly basis.	4. The Causality Assessment Sub-Committee of the National AEFI Committee conducts Causality Assessment and shares with Ministry of Health and Welfare, CDSCO and PvPI.	4. Drug Inspector (Deputed by State Drugs Control Department), CDSCO Zonal Officer under whose jurisdiction AEFI occurred, take part in joint investigation along with DIO.
		5. It is responsible for taking appropriate regulatory decisions and action on the basis of recommendations of PvPI and AEFI Secretariat.

b. *Responsibilities of Immunization Service Providers:* The surveillance of AEFI is started in 1981 in India with aim of reducing morbidity and mortality due to AEFI and minimise the negative impact of AEFI in public health. The vaccination is done at different levels and the responsibilities of the various levels of service point / service providers are:

i. Community Level (Anganwadi and ASHA / Volunteers / Front Line Workers):

    a. Doing follow up of the vaccination beneficiaries from the List of ANM and Identifying AEFIs;

    b. Informing the adverse events immediately by telephone to the concerned ANM / Medical Officer;

    c. Assisting in referral of any suspected case;

    d. Assisting the team investigating the event; and

    e. Supporting in building community confidence in immunization.

ii. Sub Centre Level:

    A. The ANM needs to note down the details of vaccines prior to use at vaccination site. The functions of ANM are:

a. Ensuring that the vaccine vial septum has not been submerged in water or contaminated;

b. Providing a list of children vaccinated to workforce at community level for follow up;

c. Entering the drop out cases with reasons in the immunization card counter foils;

d. Treating minor or non-serious AEFIs (mild symptoms like fever) symptomatically;

e. Providing immediate first aid for severe and serious adverse events and referring AEFIs to Medical Officers or to appropriate health facility for prompt treatment and report. The Medical Officer needs to be informed by the fastest means available;

f. Sharing the details of all AEFIs with Medical Officer in charge in the weekly block level meeting. It is necessary to ensure that all AEFIs are entered in the AEFI register; and

g. Assisting the investigation of AEFIs and taking initiative for corrective action on advice of Medical Officer.

B. Health Supervisors:

a. Supervising and providing hands on training to the ANMs and other vaccinators;

b. Monitoring the community for adverse events during supervisory visit to immunization site / service centres;

c. Encouraging the health workers to report AEFIs and emphasizing the need of immediate notification of serious / severe AEFIs;

d. Analysing the reported AEFIs in Sub Centre's monthly report and tracking of health workers who have not reported any AEFI over a period of time; and

e. Assisting the investigating team in conducting the investigation.

iii. Block PHC / CHC /Corporation / Ward / Urban Health Post level (Medical Officer in Charge):

a. Training staff in detecting, managing and reporting AEFIs and differentiating between minor and serious / severe events;

b. Encouraging the staff to report AEFIs;

c. Enquiring about any recent outbreak of disease or illness or ant death in the community which may or may not have been related to vaccination;

d. Ensuring clinical case management of AEFIs and referring to the next level facility if needed;

e. Ensuring availability of emergency drugs and equipments to deal with an adverse event;

f. Regularly checking functional status of equipments and expiry of drugs; and

g. Ensuring the familiarity of ANMs with the use of anaphylaxis kit.

iv. Private Sector: Private sectors contribute significantly in immunization coverage both in rural and urban India. The private sector immunization providers are encouraged to report the AEFI incidents using CRF to the nearest government health facility or DIO. The Indian Association of Paediatricians has a software for reporting infectious diseases and this has provision for reporting AEFI.

v. District Level: The District Immunization Officer or Chief Medical Officer is entrusted with managing AEFI at district level:

a. Establishing functional AEFI Committeeand maintenance of documentation of AEFI activities;

b. Maintaining the list of non-investigated reported cases of serious / severe and minor AEFI and inform the AEFI Committee in next meeting for further action;

c. Coordinating with PvPI's ADR monitoring centre to ensure the identified ADRs following vaccination are reported to DIO;

d. Coordinating with Medical Colleges identifying the expertise who would help the committee in investigating the case;

e. Building relationship with local chapters of IMA /IAP; share personal contact details with all concerned persons for prompt reporting;

f. Ensuring availability of adequate reporting forms and logistics such as Auto Destructive Syringes to prevent AEFI due to programme errors;

g. Ensuring dissemination of AEFI guidelines and training of staff to detect and report adverse events in time;

h. Receiving and analysing AEFIs reported through various sources; and discuss the same at monthly Medical officers' meeting;

i. Completing the CRF and sharing the form with State and National level functionaries within 24 hours of submission by Medical officer;

j. Ensuring all serious / severe AEFI in coordination with the District Committee at the earliest;

k. Ensuring timely management of all cases in the district; and

l. Sending CRFs and CIFs from the district to state EPI officer and national immunization division.

vi. State Level: Director of Family Welfare / State Immunization Officer and State Drugs Controller are responsible for:

a. Coordinating and leading AEFI activities in the state;

b. Establishing functional AEFI committee (this includes state drugs controller) and maintaining AEFI related documentation;

c. Ensuring periodic training and dissemination of AEFI guidelines and reporting forms to all concerned persons;

d. Assisting in responding to AEFI and supporting the districts in investigation;

e. Reviewing the key updates in the monthly meeting of state task force on immunization;

f. Ensuring the availability of updated list of ADR monitoring centre to the DIOs;

g. Coordinating with sate chapters of IMA / IAP to ensure reporting by private practitioners from the districts;

h. Ensuring AEFI monitoring and supporting supervision;

i.   Coordinating with medical colleges for support in investigating AEFI cases;

j.   Receiving and analysing reported AEFIs and sharing feedback with central government and districts;

k.   Monitoring reported data for detection of previously unrecognised potential signals out of vaccine related adverse events and make recommendation for further investigation;

l.   Reviewing AEFI cases during state and district review meeting and workshops;

m.   Providing feedback of observations and recommendations of the state AEFI committee and specimen testing results to the concerned DIO;

n.   Reviewing the data whether similar events have occurred in other districts; coordinating with DIOs and providing technical assistance if required;

o.   Coordinating with other state departments to deal with any referral or testing need following AEFIs;

p.   Conducting quality causality assessments of each reported case at the state level within 100 days of notification of AEFI cases; and

q.   Ensuring submission of all documents including hospital records and post-mortem reports by the districts.

c. *Responsibilities of Marketing Authorization Holders (MAH)of Vaccines:*

i.   The MAH should have a PV system in place for collecting, processing and forwarding the reports on AEFI arise from the use of vaccine manufactured (or imported) and marketed in India. The reports should be forwarded to the Licencing Authority. The system needs to be managed by a medical officer or pharmacist trained in collection and analysis of ADRs (Designated Person). The MAH is responsible for appropriate action, whenever a safety issue arises, after due investigation and scientific evaluation. When PV activities are carried out by a third party, a contractual agreement describing responsibilities of each must be in place;

ii.   The Designated Person is responsible for submitting domestic serious and unexpected ADRs, foreign serious unexpected

ADRs, and any follow up information after initial case reports to the CDSCO within 15 days of receipt;

iii. Designated Person is responsible for submitting PSUR as required by the Licencing Authority. The PSUR is usually required to be submitted every six months for the first two years and then annually for next two years after receiving marketing authorization,

iv. The Designated Person needs to conduct critical analysis of ADR reports received and prepare summary report on annual basis or as required by the Licensing Authorities of Central and State Government;

v. The Designated Person should periodically perform literature search and report the findings to the Licensing Authority; and

vi. The MAH should arrange periodic self-inspection by the person independent of PV system and initiate corrective actions.

Issues of vaccine Hesitancy: There are many controversies associated with the use of vaccines which led to reduced vaccine acceptance and decreased vaccine coverage leading to increase in vaccine preventable diseases. One of the classic example is: Vaccine causing autism - 'The measles, mumps and rubella vaccine might cause autism' was first reported in 1998 in the prestigious Lancet. The article received intense media and public attention; and perhaps caused maximum damage to the vaccination programme. The article was later retracted because of improprieties in subject recruitment and financial conflict of interest. Though many studies have arguable concluded that there is no association between the MMR vaccination and autism, peoples' perception has not changed completely. There are other examples too: Mercury (preservative) content of vaccine causes neurodevelopmental disorder; Vaccines cause Guillain – Barre Syndrome (GBS); and Vaccine causes autoimmune illness. Polio vaccination is a foreign ploy to sterilize Muslims. In India too there was large scale misconception: polio vaccine causes impotency was wide spread in some communities in India. The World Health Organization has recently identified "Refusal or hesitation to get vaccination against the deadly diseases despite availability of effective vaccines" as one of the top ten threats to global health for 2019.

Vaccine hesitancy is a complex issue and one single strategy will not be helpful globally. But the vaccine surveillance is a way to restore public confidence.

Key Messages

- The safety monitoring of vaccines is essential like that of other medicinal products.

  The vaccine pharmacovigilance is defined as the science and activities relating to detection, assessment, understanding, prevention and communication of adverse events following immunization or any other vaccine or immunization related issues. The adverse event monitoring programme of vaccine is known as 'Adverse Event Following Immunization (AEFI)'

- AEFIs are very critical as misconceptions about vaccine safety can completely destroy the Immunization programme. Vaccine hesitancy arise out of misconception is one of the top 10 public health threat.

- The AEFIs are classified into four types: Vaccine Reactions – cause specific reactions, vaccine reactions by seriousness and frequency; immunization errorrelated reactions – handling error in vaccine / diluent, prescribing error / non-adherence to recommendation, administration error; immunization anxiety related reactions; and coincidental events.

- Causality assessment of AEFIs helps in identification of vaccine related problems; identification of immunization related problems; excluding coincidental events; detection of potential signals; and validation of pre-licensure safety data.

- On causality analysis, AEFI cases are classified into four categories: A (consistent causal association to immunization); B (indeterminate); C (coincidental or inconsistent causal association with immunization); and D (unclassifiable).

- At all service providing points: Community level, Sub-Centre level, Block Level and District level, the service providers are responsible to detect and report AEFI. At District level there is District AEFI committee and at State Level State AEFI Committee. The State Immunization Officer is responsible for submitting the AEFI details to the Central Government.

- National Pharmacovigilance Coordination Centre (PvPI), AEFI Secretariat, and CDSCO work in coordination with each other ensuring vaccine safety.

- The Marketing Authorization Holder is responsible to establish PV system and appoints a designated person to oversee the PV activities including submission of reports. The designated person is either a doctor or pharmacist with training on PV.

Bibliography

1. Adverse Events Following Immunization - Surveillance and Response Operational Guidelines, MOHFW, 2015.

2. AEFI Surveillance and Response, Operational Guidelines, Government of India, 2010.

3. Causality assessment of an adverse event following immunization (AEFI): user manual for the revised WHO classification (Second edition). Geneva: World Health Organization; 2018.

4. GP Mohanta, RT Saravanakumar and PK Manna, Vaccine hesitation – a threat to global health. *Chronicle Pharmabiz, Vol. 19 (32), page 10, July 10, 2019.*

5. Guidance for Industry on Pharmacovigilance Requirements for Biological Products, Central Drugs Standard Control Organization, Ministry of Health and Family Welfare, Government of India, 2017.

6. Immunization Handbook for Medical Officers, Department of Health and Family Welfare, Government of India, 2008.

7. Scott C. Ratzan *et al, Salzburg Statement on Vaccine Acceptance,* Journal of Health Communication, 0: 1–3, 2019.

Chapter 16

Case Studies on Drugs Withdrawal

"If you look over a list of medicinal recipe in vogue in the last century, how foolish and useless they are seem to be! And yet we use equally absurd ones with faith today".

Henry David Thoreau

Thalidomide: the Greatest Drug Disaster

Thalidomide is perhaps one of the greatest drug tragedies that has changed the course of safety monitoring (Pharmacovigilance) system in the world. The drug was synthesized in 1956 by a German company, Chemie. The invention of thalidomide was a new venture for the company which used to make cosmetics and household products. The company had little or no experience on pharmaceuticals. Thalidomide showed considerable promise as a sleeping tablet and as an alternative to barbiturate. It had better safety profile than barbiturate as overdosing 100 times the normal dose was not lethal. Besides, it did not have the risk of 'hangover' effects that might affect driving or operating heavy machineries.

The company started marketing thalidomide in Germany in October 1957 under the name of Contergan. Its equivalent Distaval was marketed in England. It was hailed as "tranquiliser of the future". Within a year of thalidomide's introduction in Germany, an extremely rare birth deformity began to appear. Babies were born with short, finlike flaps instead of normal arms and legs. It was in November 1961, a German paediatrician declared that the outbreak of this gross malformation, phocomelia, to the use in the pregnancy of the new hypnotic drug. In 1961 December, the first report of association was published in a widely circulated medical journal indicating that thalidomide might be human teratogen. The number of cases of phocomelia had mysteriously increased from 12 in 1959, to 83 in 1960, to 360 in 1961 in Germany alone. It was estimated that more than 10,000 babies of twenty countries were the victim of thalidomide. Of these, around 50% (5000) survived and 1600 of whom eventually needed artificial limbs. The drug was finally withdrawn in 1961.

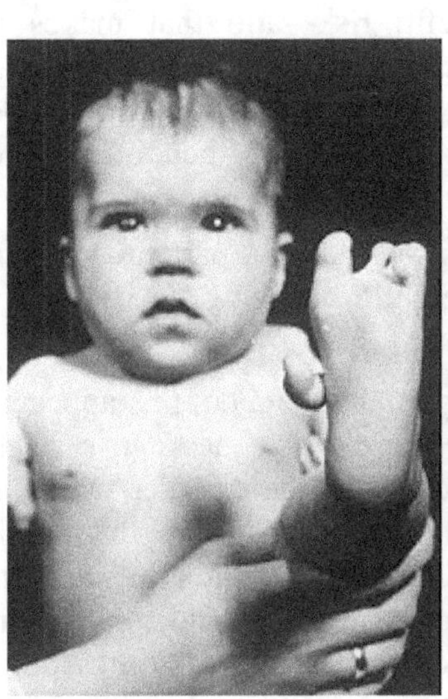 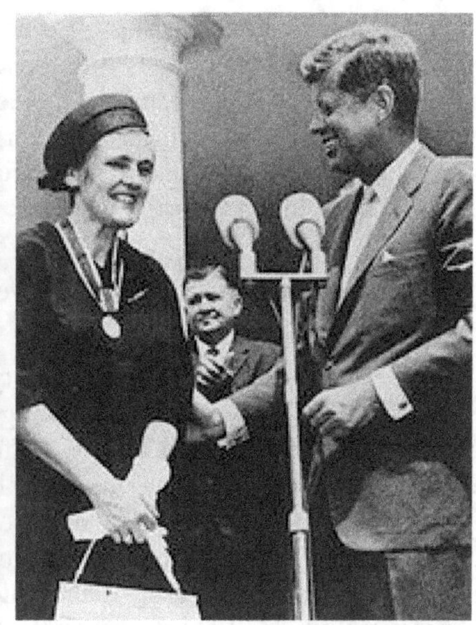

In 1960, a US pharmaceutical company, Merrell Pharmaceuticals, applied for permission to market in USA. By this time many countries had permitted its use. In October 1961, the newly joined medical officer, Dr. (Ms.) Frances Kelsey, was assigned the task of supervising the approval process of thalidomide. At that time, USFDA had to reject the approval within 60 days or automatically allow marketing. Though the company was eagerly waiting for its approval, Kelsey kept on stalling after each 60 days period rejecting the application incomplete. She was apprehensive of some data: one of the side effects was mild neuritis or tingling of nerves. She was trying to correlate her research of fifteen years before that the neuritis of this type in pregnant animals resulted in deformed offspring. She was just waiting for little longer before making a decision which paid. Then of course, the non-lethal but shocking adverse effect of thalidomide was known to the world. While the children of more than 20 countries including UK, Australia, Belgium, Switzerland, were affected by this thalidomide, FDA medical officer, Kelsey saved the America by her heroic 'no' to thalidomide despite pressure. In 1962, Dr. Frances Kelsey was awarded the President's Gold Medal for distinguished service.

A review of the experimental work carried out with thalidomide before marketing revealed that inappropriate toxicological data had been published and animal findings were misinterpreted. Thalidomide disaster had taught many lessons and is also classic example to cite:

- A clear understanding of benefit and risk: No medicine is absolutely safe. It is the benefit: risk ratio that makes the usefulness of substance as medicine. Thalidomide has now made a comeback as drug for refractory multiple myeloma and leprosy. In these patients, it outweighs risk in favour of benefit, provided it is not given to fertile women.

- It is not that everyone is at the same risk of a particular adverse effect. Women who do not have child bearing capacity have no risk at all.

In spite of so much negative publicity of thalidomide, this appears to be still used for nausea and alleviating morning sickness. In a related case, one petitioner alleged that he suffers from the disorder which has affected two fingers each on both his hands due to thalidomide prescription to mother. Bombay High Court has asked the Food and Drug Administration (FDA) to consider issuing a circular for doctors pointing out the side effects of the drug 'thalidomide'. [Source: http://drugscontrol. org/news.asp?id=8749&hl=Consider%20issuing%20circular%20on%20si de-effects%20of%20drug:%20HC%20to%20FDA, accessed on 15 October 2013].

Bibliography

1. Bill Inman, Don't tell the patient, Highland Park Production, USA, 1999.

2. Charles F. Levinthal, Drugs, Behavior, and Modern Society, Second Edition, Allyn and Bacon, USA, 1999.

3. Mohanta, G.P., P.K. Manna, and R. Manavalan. "Drug Tragedies-A Review." Indian Journal of Pharmaceutical Education, 35.2 (2001): 65-66.

Diethylstilbestrol – Once a Popular Remedy only with Risk without Benefit!

The drug was promoted as a preventive measure for miscarriage based on the theory that habitual abortion was caused due to lack of progesterone and could be prevented by giving oestrogen that would in turn stimulate the production of progesterone. Based on this just theory, it was prescribed to millions of patients worldwide over 30 years and was stopped when it was found to cause cancer. This is diethylstilbestrol (DES). This was three times more potent than natural oestrogen. Though the use of DES has been discontinued since early 1970s, its impact on DES children continues! It has been described as a toxic time bomb referring to the long gestation period for the side effects to emerge and the effects may even stretch into third generations. The adverse effects was not only restricted to the user, the women during pregnancy, but has been percolated to the sons and daughters of the user.

DES, a first synthetic female hormone (oestrogen), was developed by Sir Edward Charles Dodds in 1938. He was a British Biochemist and was looking for synthetic oestrogens that could be easily and inexpensively made to treat symptoms of menopause. The beauty of DES was that it can be taken orally unlike the natural oestrogen and was not patented. The several pharmaceutical companies across the globe exploited this molecule and promoted for preventing abortion, miscarriage, premature labour and for several other conditions. In USA alone 267 pharmaceutical companies sold DES. A poorly designed study of 632 pregnant women reported in 1948 "the administration of DES could increase the chance of successful in women who had previous miscarriage or suffered from high blood pressure and risk of premature deliveries would be avoided". This has further promoted the prescription of DES.

The animal studies between 1930 and 1940 showed that DES and other oestrogens could cause cancer. The clinical studies proved its ineffectiveness. A randomised controlled trial involving 1600 women reported in 1953 showed that DES did not reduce the incidence of abortion, prematurity or post maturity. However, it was claimed that the investigators failed to report its adverse effects or risks from the study data. The study data showed significant increased abortion, neonatal deaths and premature births. Though animal studies showed the link between DES and cancer earlier, the link in humans was found only in 1971. The research showed a rare form of vaginal and cervical cancer in daughters of women who had taken DES early in pregnancy. It was found in the women in their early twenties. DES effect was termed as medically used disease. Following these reports, the US FDA in 1971 advised the physicians to discontinue prescribing DES to pregnant women. Other countries reacted slowly. Its use in pregnancy continued in France till 1977.

The DES was never banned but its indication in pregnancy was only withdrawn. Its use continued for the treatment of advanced prostate cancer, advanced breast cancer in post menopausal women, inhibition of lactation, amenorrhoea, vaginal irritation and morning after pill (post coital contraceptive). The use of DES in USA was continued till 1997. The DES was also promoted in veterinary practice as growth stimulant. People taking these animal foods were also exposed to the effects of DES. The DES is currently in use for the treatment of breast cancer and prostate cancer.

The DES was not only ineffective for the purpose for which it was promoted, it caused several adverse effects including impacting at least three generations. It had caused cell adenocarcinoma, a rare cancer in DES daughters (daughters of mothers taken DES during pregnancy). The risk is rare and range from one in 1000 to one in 10,000 exposed daughters. In addition, there were other risks: DES daughters were at twice risk to develop pre-cancerous abnormalities of the cervix, vagina and carcinoma in situ; development of adenosis (more abundant vaginal discharge); development of structural defects of cervix, vagina, uterus, fallopian tubes; more likely to be infertile; increased risk of adverse pregnancy outcomes; four time the risk of miscarriage and preterm labour; and the more chances of life threatening ectopic pregnancy. The DES sons too have their share of risk like increase in epididymal and testicular abnormalities such as undescended testes, incomplete or defective testicular developments and low sperm counts.

It has been estimated that a large number of women worldwide were exposed to action of DES: 20 to 30 lakh in USA, 40 lakh in Canada, 40 lakh in Europe, 2 lakh in France and 10 thousand in Australia. Realising the long term impact of DES use, the authorities advised the DES daughters to undergo annual cytological screening and colposcopic examination of both the cervix and vagina. The DES daughters of above 40 are advised annual mammography.

Many lawsuits have been filed in different parts of the world claiming compensation for the victims of DES. As there were large number of brands and considerable time is lapsed, it was difficult for the people to recollect the brand or company. In 1980, California Supreme Court ruled that the women should be able to fight as a group and the companies are liable to pay based on their market share. In a similar judgement in 1992, the Dutch Supreme Court ruled that every manufacturer should be equally and fully liable for damages, regardless of their market share at that time. In one judgement (2012) ordered 14 pharmaceutical companies to negotiate compensation for 53 women who alleged that their breast cancer was caused by their mothers' use of DES a decade ago. Perhaps the first settlement between four sisters and the Eli Lily has been reached in early 2013. It was alleged that the company did not test the drug adequately before marketing.

The use of DES though thought to be safe and effective, it was proved otherwise. The administration of any oestrogen is contraindicated during pregnancy. Its complete adverse effects are not yet known. As it is expected to harm even the third generation, we need to wait for the time when the youngest DES daughters reach the age of menopause perhaps by 2040. The DES is one of the greatest drug disasters but little focussed on its tragic effects.

Bibliography

1. British National Formulary (63), March 2012.

2. Chetly, A., The time bomb explodes in Problem Drugs, Health Action International, 1993.

3. DES Update Home, http://www.cdc.gov/des/index.html accessed on 07 December 2013.

4. Diethylstilboestrol (DES) Exposure in Utero, College Statement of The Royal Australian and New Zealand College of Obstetricians and Gynaecologists, March 2013.

5. Martindale: The Complete Drug Reference, Thirty fourth edition, Pharmaceutical Press, 2005.

Rofecoxib (Vioxx) – Association with Serious Cardiovascular Events

The harm caused by the use of Rofecoxib is regarded the single greatest drug safety catastrophe in USA and possibly in the history of the world. It was believed that this could have been largely or completely avoided. A senior US FDA officer testified that it might have caused more than 1, 00,000 heart attacks and strokes including an estimated 40,000 deaths. The drug was withdrawn by the innovator company in 2004 just after five years of use.

Rofecoxib was introduced in US market by Merck in 1999 with the brand name vioxx as an effective and safer alternative to NSAIDs for the treatment of pain associated with osteoarthritis. Rofecoxib is the selective cyclooxygenase -2 (COX-2) inhibitor. It was believed that selective inhibition of COX-2 enzyme would provide relief from pain and inflammation. As it does not interfere in COX-1, the production of COX-1 would remain and protect the gastrointestinal tract. The traditional NSAIDs provide relief from pain and inflammation through reducing the production of prostaglandin. Prostaglandins are produced at the site of injury and inflammation thus reduction of these provide anti-inflammatory effects. Prostaglandins do help protecting the stomach lining from acidic effect of gastric fluid. The traditional NSAIDs inhibit both the COX – 1 and COX – 2 enzymes and reduce the prostaglandin synthesis and thus provide anti-inflammatory effects and have long been associated with increased risk of gastrointestinal perforation, ulcers and bleeding. Thus the selective COX- 2 inhibitor, Rofecoxib, was termed as the miracle drug.

In reality the situation was different. The other effects of COX – 2 inhibitors were not given due importance in an attempt to conceal the safety data and promote Rofecoxib which was prescribed to more than 20 million Americans generating a revenue over USD 2 billion annually. The COX – 1 and the COX – 2 enzymes have different physiological roles. The COX – 1 produces thromboxane, a vasoconstrictor and platelet aggregator. On the other hand, COX – 2 enzyme produces prostacyclin, a vasodilator and anti-aggregating agent. Anti-aggregation of platelets and vasodilatation are important defence mechanisms for the human body when faced with onset of a cardiovascular event. Selective inhibition of COX – 2 enzyme disables this defence mechanism and the effects of COX – 1 thus puts the patients at higher risk of cardiovascular events.

The balance of COX – 1 and COX – 2 activities are disturbed. Besides, prostacyclin plays a role in the development of arteriosclerosis and in thinning of plaque along the wall of blood vessels. The particles of plaque are released due to rupture of the plaque and can cause thrombosis. This is the precise mechanism how the use of Rofecoxib was more risky in causing cardiovascular events.

Several studies reported the increased risk of cardiovascular events like increased heart attack with both low and high doses of rofecoxib use. There was even allegation that the Merck Company did know the risk but did not disclose. The company disseminated the pooled data of several small studies to promote the drug's cardiovascular safety to doctors in its cardio vascular card. The company's vioxx gastrointestinal outcomes research (VIGOR) launched in January 1999 was intended to expand the drug's approved indications comparing with naproxen for the treatment of rheumatoid arthritis. The authors withheld the critical data on cardiovascular toxicity. Its results were viewed with suspicion. Even though it was reported that the study did not follow Standard Operating Procedure (SOP), results disclosed in November 1999 showed 79% greater risk of deaths or cardiovascular events in one treatment group. A leading Medical Journal's Editor expressed that rofecoxib was not more effective than naproxen in relieving rheumatoid arthritis but did the halves the gastrointestinal risk. Another study called, APPROVe (Adenomatous Polyp Prevention on VIOXX) trial, was initiated to see if Vioxx 25 mg was effective in preventing the occurrence of colon polyps. Contrary to the expectation, the result showed an increased heart attacks and strokes after 18 months of continuous treatment compared to placebo. The study was stopped. In addition to its own research findings, the company came to know of the similar findings by USFDA, forced the Merck to withdraw its product Vioxx from the market effective 30 September 2004. There have been several legal suits. The company spent nearly $6bn as legal expense to settle vioxx related cases in USA alone. Many cases in UK and Australia too filed.

The funniest part was that its return to use was encouraged by USFDA with expanded safety warning and without advertising directly to the consumers. However, it did not return to the market. In India, the drug was manufactured and sold by several companies. The Government of India banned its use from 13 December 2004. A terrible tragedy could have been avoided had the company acted responsibly and the regulatory authority been more alert.

Bibliography

1. Andy D. Birchfield, Jr *et al,* The Vioxx Story, a Portion of Plaintiff's position Paper in MDL# 1657, 2007.

2. Harlan Krumholz *et al,* What have we learnt from Vioxx?, British Medical Journal, 334, 20 January 2007.

3. Janice Hopkins Tanne, Merck pays $ 1 bn penalty in relation to promotion of rofecoxib, British Medical Journal, 343, 28 November 2011.

4. Rofecoxib, Heart Attacks, and the FDA: Testimony of David J. Graham, November 18, 2004 (From The Revised A Lay person's Guide to Medicines, LOCOST, Vadodara, 2006).

Pioglitazone – Association with Bladder Cancer

The Government of India had suspended the manufacture, sale and distribution of popular anti-diabetic drug Pioglitazone in June 2013. But, it was subsequently reintroduced. The suspending notification claimed "the Government is satisfied that the use of drug Pioglitazone and all drug formulations containing Pioglitazone are likely to involve risk to human beings and the safer alternatives are available and hence the decision to suspend". The decision was not taken without following the standard procedure of discussion in DTAB (Drugs Technical Advisory Board) and without looking of hard evidence when the National Pharmacovigilance Programme is in place.

Pioglitazone belongs to the antidiabetic group of medicines 'thiazolidinediones (or glitazones)' was approved in US in early 1999. The two other drugs of the same glitazone group are withdrawn or severely restricted of use. Troglitazone within three years of introduction was removed because of its liver toxicity. Rosiglitazone is banned in many countries including India because of its association with elevated risk of cardiovascular events like heart attack and heart failure. In USA it is not banned but available with restricted use.

The animal studies had shown that Pioglitazone cause urinary bladder tumour in male rats in a two year study. Based on some studies US FDA in 2010 issued safety warning that there has been evidence to suggest that an increased risk of bladder cancer in patients with largest exposure of Pioglitazone and those taking highest cumulative dose. Further on 04 August 2011 warned the Healthcare Professionals and also a change in product label that the use of the drug for more than one year may be associated with increased risk of bladder cancer. It recommended "Not to use Pioglitazone in patients with active bladder cancer" and "Use with caution in patients with a prior history of bladder cancer". The FDA calculated the risk as the use of Pioglitazone was associated with 27.5 excess cases of bladder cancer per one lakh patients using the drug for one year compared to those who never use Pioglitazone.

Worst Pills, Best Pills, an independent drug information bulletin of USA termed the drug, Pioglitazone, as do not use category drug. It advised the patients not to use this antidiabetic drug as it is associated with several other side effects like liver damage, weight gain, anaemia and heart failure in addition to the risk of bladder cancer. The safer alternatives like glimepiride, glipizide, glyburide, tolazamide, tolbuta-mide and metformin.

France had suspended the use of Pioglitazone and Germany recommended that no new patients be given Pioglitazone. Though there has been perceived of a potential safety risk there is no established causal relationship between the use of Pioglitazone and bladder cancer.

Pioglitazone with respect to Bladder Cancer [Source: PvPI Newsletter, August 2013 Issue]	
Country	**Regulatory Status**
India	The drug should not be used as first line therapy of diabetes. The manufacturers should mention box warning in bold red letters.
France	Banned in July 2011
United States	Label Warning like 'not to use in patients with active bladder cancer'.
Japan	Label Warning like 'not to use in patients with active bladder cancer'.
Germany	Label warning like 'due to slight increase of risk bladder cancer the doctors should not prescribe in patients with bladder cancer (visible blood in the urine'.
There were reports of 54 ADRs for the drug in Indian database comprising of facial oedema, hypoglycaemia, aggravated hypoglycaemia, oedema, oedema in legs, giddiness, hypotension and drowsiness. There was only one case of bladder carcinoma in Indian database against the reports of 1241 cases globally as of June 2013.	

In India, the Government of India, Ministry of Health and Family Welfare (CDSCO)'s ban was misfired inviting protests from all over. Finally, the Government tracked back 'it is re-looking at the whole issue'. The decision to notification suspending the use of the drug was issued without following the standard protocol. The Ministry had not consulted the highest technical body, DTAB and was the unilateral whimsical decision of the country's top drug regulatory body, central drugs standard control organization.

Millions of diabetic patients are with pioglitazone, a cost effective medicine. The sudden banning of the medicine causes not only panic but also inconvenience to the patient as well to doctors. The medicine is not only regulates the blood glucose level but has additional advantages of regulating triglyceride level. It seems eight cases of bladder cancer in patients with pioglitazone were observed and the case reports were published in a journal as the letter to the editor. This report is not as peer reviewed scientific publication. While the millions of patients are under pioglitazone, it is not known the observations of 8 cases are out of how many?? This was one of the issues in the controversial ban.

On review of the decision, Drugs and Technical Advisory Board (DTAB), recommended the continuing use of pioglitazone but with a warning. DTAB is the highest advisory board of experts that recommends the government on technical matters relating to medicines. Similar to the US warning, now it is recommended to restrict the dose to 30 mg and screening of patients every six months for side effects.

In an interesting incidence, the Japanese Pharmaceutical Company, Takeda, agreed to pay up to $2.4 billion to settle US suits against its actos (pioglitazone). It was alleged that it hid the cancer risk of the drug. Though the company seems to have not agreed to the allegation but went for out of court settlement as strategy to 'reduce financial uncertainties'. [Source: News Reports of 28th April 2015 appeared in various media].

Bibliography

1. Bladder Cancer Warning for Pioglitazone, Worst Pills Best Pills Newsletter, November 2011.

2. GSR 379 (E), Ministry of Health and Family Welfare, 18 June 2013, The Gazette of India, New Delhi No. 294, June 18, 2013.

3. GSR 520 (E), Ministry of Health and Family Welfare, 31 July 2013, The Gazette of India, New Delhi No. 384, July 31, 2013.

4. Guru Prasad Mohanta, Much ado, nothing? Orissa Post, 09 August 2013.

5. Guru Prasad Mohanta, Pioglitazone: Unneeded Controversy, The Pharma Review, May – June 2014.

6. Hashmi A., Pioglitazone suspension and its aftermath: A wake up call for the Indian drug regulatory authorities, J Pharmacol Pharmacother, 2013.

7. R. Prasad, Diabetes drug: 'May be I erred in my judgement', The Hindu, 17th July 2013.

Chapter 17

Case Studies on Causality Assessment

"Tell me and I will forget, Show me and I will remember, Involve me and I will understand".

Confucius

CASE STUDY – 1 [Certain]

Mr. G, 42 year old, was admitted in surgery ward after haemorrhoidectomy. He was known allergic to Aspirin, Paracetamol and Diclofenac. Patient had no known comorbidity at the time of surgery.

His treating surgeon decided to put him on Inj Cefaperazone + Sulbactum 1.5 g q12h and Inj Metronidazole 0.5 g q12h; and Inj Ketorolac. Cefaperazone, Sulbactum and Metronidazole were meant for preventing post surgical infection and Ketorolac for the management of post operative pain. Prior to IV administration, test dose of Ketorolac was given intradermally to rule out allergic reactions, if any, and was put on observation for 30 minutes. Patient was found to be normal with no signs of allergic reaction. Following the test for allergic reaction, he was administered Ketorolac. .

Following Inj Ketorolac 30 mg IV infusion, within 15 minutes patient started developing erythema on face which soon progressed to upper limbs and trunk followed by periorbital oedema, dyspnoea and hypotension (BP = 80/60 mmHg). The infusion was immediately stopped following which gradual symptomatic improvement was noticed.

Clinician made an impression about the reaction as acute anaphylaxis. Assess the causality for the given reaction using Naranjo's Probability Scale and explain.

S. No.	Questions	Yes	No	Don't know	Score
1	Are there previous *conclusive* reports on this reaction?	+1	0	0	+1
2	Did the adverse event appear after the suspected drug was administered?	+2	-1	0	+2
3	Did the adverse reaction improve when the drug was discontinued or a *specific* antagonist was administered?	+1	0	0	+1
4	Did the adverse event reappear when the drug was re-administered?	+2	-1	0	0
5	Are there alternative causes (other than the drug) that could on their own have caused the reaction?	-1	+2	0	+2
6	Did the reaction reappear when a placebo was given?	-1	+1	0	0
7	Was the drug detected in blood (or other fluids) in concentrations known to be toxic?	+1	0	0	0
8	Was the reaction more severe when the dose was increased or less severe when the dose was decreased?	+1	0	0	0
9	Did the patient have a similar reaction to the same or similar drugs in *any* previous exposure?	+1	0	0	+1
10	Was the adverse event confirmed by any objective evidence?	+1	0	0	+1
	TOTAL SCORE				+8

This patient was known allergic to multiple drugs and had high risk in developing reaction with similar class of drugs as mentioned above. He had no other medically relevant co-morbidity. The reaction was clinically (objective) evident, had obvious and plausible time relationship with medication administered. IV infusion of ketorolac was stopped immediately after onset of reaction and the patient started recovering gradually within an hour after infusion was stopped.

Item no. 4 and 6 have been assigned 0 indicating don't know (note that don't know is to be used sparingly, here it denotes not applicable). Total score is +8 using Naranjo scale but Anaphylaxis falls in special category of causality where usual parameter like rechallenge is not applicable. In this case suspected drug was given in the form IV infusion and therefore dechallenge can be applied. Remember that Rechallenge is never done in serious reactions like this in the interest of patient safety (it is unethical too). Causality for anaphylaxis is always assessed as ***Certain.***

Using WHO scale for this example

*(Consider the points written in **bold** while working with WHO scale).*

Patient did not show any sign of reaction with test dose but with full dose. There is obvious and **reasonable time relationship** with drug intake and the reaction. It is **less likely** to be **attributed** to **disease** and the **other concomitant drug** as well. But ketorolac is highly suspected because patient has history of reaction for similar drugs and reaction **(anaphylaxis)** occurred within 15 minutes while on ketorolac. Only because patient was on IV infusion drug was stopped. Correlating all these data in the given case, the given example falls under the category ***"Certain" (special category).***

CASE STUDY – 2 [Certain]

A 31 year old fisherwoman weighing 49 kg, a known case of Pulmonary Tuberculosis, was with regimen CAT II ATT (oral Isoniazid 300 mg, Rifampicin 450 mg, Pyrazinamide 1500 mg, Ethambutol 1200 mg and inj Streptomycin 750 mg) since 15/01/15. She was neither receiving any concomitant drugs nor had any known co-morbidity. Family history of lymph node TB is known in her sister and brother. On 30/01/15 she came to dermatology OPD having developed generalized itching and rashes all over the body including face, numbness and swelling of lips. Patient was immediately admitted suspecting an ATT drugs induced ADR. She was symptomatically treated with Inj Avil and calamine lotion. On 4/02/15 she was symptomatically better and stable hence the physician decided to restart individual ATT drugs (same dose and brand was administered) considering her medical condition. It was found that the patient tolerated Isoniazid and Rifampicin but she developed generalized rash and itching all over the body within 2 hours following oral Pyrazinamide and dizziness, numbness, swelling of lips following inj Streptomycin. This time reaction was more severe than previous episode. Hence *clinician made an impression that patient is allergic to Pyrazinamide and Streptomycin*. Offending drugs were stopped and patient was put on modified ATT drug regimen.

(*Note*: ATT means anti-tubercular treatment; CAT stands for Category)

Assess the causality for the given reaction using Naranjo's Probability Scale and explain.

S. No.	Questions	Yes	No	Don't know	Score
1	Are there previous *conclusive* reports on this reaction?	+1	0	0	+1
2	Did the adverse event appear after the suspected drug was administered?	+2	-1	0	+2
3	Did the adverse reaction improved when the drug was discontinued or a *specific* antagonist was administered?	+1	0	0	+1
4	Did the adverse event reappear when the drug was re-administered?	+2	-1	0	+2
5	Are there alternative causes (other than the drug) that could on their own have caused the reaction?	-1	+2	0	+2
6	Did the reaction reappear when a placebo was given?	-1	+1	0	0
7	Was the drug detected in blood (or other fluids) in concentrations known to be toxic?	+1	0	0	0
8	Was the reaction more severe when the dose was increased or less severe when the dose was decreased?	+1	0	0	+1
9	Did the patient have a similar reaction to the same or similar drugs in *any* previous exposure?	+1	0	0	0
10	Was the adverse event confirmed by any objective evidence?	+1	0	0	+1
	TOTAL SCORE				+10

The event was clinically specific and date of drug administration and onset of reaction had plausible time relationship. Patient was not on any concomitant drugs. Dechallenge is considered positive since patient recovered symptomatically in five days after withdrawal of the suspected drug. Rechallenge was done using one drug at a time to identify the culprit drug/s. It was found that following administration of Pyrazinamide as well as Streptomycin reactions reappeared and that they were more severe than the previous episode. Therefore, it was confirmed that the offending agents were Pyrazinamide and Streptomycin.

As the total score is +10, the causality is attributed as **Certain**.

[Always remember, "**Rechallenge**" means same drug, brand, dose and frequency. If not it is categorized as "reintroduction" and therefore assessment may change to ***Probable.***]

*Using **WHO** scale for this example*

*(Consider the points in **Bold** while working with WHO scale).*

In the above case, there is **plausible time relationship** with drug intake and reaction. There is **no correlation** with the disease and both **dechallenge** and **rechallenge** are positive for pyrazinamide and streptomycin; therefore, assessed as *"Certain"*

CASE STUDY – 3 [Probable]

A 65 year old female patient, a known case of COPD for last four years, was admitted in medicine wing of hospital with complaint of severe acute bronchospasm. Her weight was 58 kg. She was not known to have any drug allergy.

She was given the following medications after admission:

- Nebulizer Salbutamol 2.5 mg q6h
- Inj Aminophylline 300 mg dissolved in 20 ml of 5% dextrose over 20 minutes
- Inj Ampicillin 1g q6h
- Inj Furosemide 40 mg IV BD (last dose to be given by 4 pm)

At night 8 pm a duty physician observed disorientation and drowsiness in patient and he immediately ordered tests for serum electrolytes. The laboratory report showed a decreased levels of Sodium and Potassium: Serum Na^+ =114 mmol/L, Serum K^+=2.9 mmol/L. Physician suspected it to be **drug induced hyponatremia and hypokalemia due to Inj Furosemide;** thereby, the patient was given Inj. Potassium chloride. Additionally high salt in diet was also advised. (Note that the drug was not withdrawn considering furosemide as first line drug for peripheral oedema in COPD patients). After 7 days, serum electrolytes returned to normal levels (Serum Na^+=135 mmol/L, Serum K^+=3.8 mmol/L). Therefore, patient recovered.

Assess the causality for the given reaction using Naranjo's Probability Scale and explain.

S. No.	Questions	Yes	No	Don't know	Score
1	Are there previous *conclusive* reports on this reaction?	+1	0	0	+1
2	Did the adverse event appear after the suspected drug was administered?	+2	-1	0	+2
3	Did the adverse reaction improve when the drug was discontinued or a *specific* antagonist was administered?	+1	0	0	+1
4	Did the adverse event reappear when the drug was re-administered?	+2	-1	0	0
5	Are there alternative causes (other than the drug) that could on their own have caused the reaction?	-1	+2	0	+2
6	Did the reaction reappear when a placebo was given?	-1	+1	0	0
7	Was the drug detected in blood (or other fluids) in concentrations known to be toxic?	+1	0	0	0
8	Was the reaction more severe when the dose was increased or less severe when the dose was decreased?	+1	0	0	0
9	Did the patient have a similar reaction to the same or similar drugs in *any* previous exposure?	+1	0	0	0
10	Was the adverse event confirmed by any objective evidence?	+1	0	0	+1
	TOTAL SCORE				+7

Patient was on various concomitant drugs but the reaction was more specific to Furosemide due to its pharmacological action. Suspected drug was not withdrawn considering critical condition of patient but Dechallenge is considered positive as patient recovered symptomatically in 7 days after intervention (Inj. Potassium chloride and additional high salt in diet).

As Naranjo's algorithm score sums to +7, its causality category is "Probable".

*Using **WHO** scale for this example*

(Consider the points in bold while working with WHO scale).

It's found that there is **fluctuation in lab data** with a **reasonable time relationship** with drug intake. The reaction is **less likely** to be attributed to disease as well. Also in this case, drug was not withdrawn considering it as important in the patient treatment regimen, but the **reaction was treated** for which patient responded positively which also means that **dechallenge is positive**. Correlating all these data in the given case, the given example falls under the category *"Probable"*.

Case Study – 4 [Probable]

A 51 year old male patient has been recently diagnosed with Rheumatoid Arthritis. His clinician put him on oral sulfasalazine 500 mg, since 09/1/15. Along with that oral methyl prednisolone 4 mg was also added to the regimen. Fifteen days later (23/01/15) the patient was brought to the emergency ward having developed generalized exanthematous rash, maculopapular in nature, red raised lesions associated with intermittent episodes of fever. On examination, the patient was also found to have hepatomegaly. His laboratory tests showed elevated levels of ALP (346 IU/L) and AEC (380 cells/cumm). Immediately drug sulfasalazine was stopped and the reactions were treated symptomatically. The patient recovered on 31/1/15 and was discharged with Methotrexate replacing sulfasalazine. He was called again after 15 days for a review and found to be well tolerating the current regimen.

[ALP= Alkaline Phosphatase, AEC= Absolute Eosinophil Count]

Clinician made an impression as drug hypersensitivity syndrome due to sulfasalazine. Assess the causality for the given reaction using Naranjo's Probability Scale and explain.

S. No.	Questions	Yes	No	Don't know	Score
1	Are there previous *conclusive* reports on this reaction?	+1	0	0	+1
2	Did the adverse event appear after the suspected drug was administered?	+2	-1	0	+2
3	Did the adverse reaction improve when the drug was discontinued or a *specific* antagonist was administered?	+1	0	0	+1
4	Did the adverse event reappear when the drug was re-administered?	+2	-1	0	0
5	Are there alternative causes (other than the drug) that could on their own have caused the reaction?	-1	+2	0	+2

Contd…

S. No.	Questions	Yes	No	Don't know	Score
6	Did the reaction reappear when a placebo was given?	-1	+1	0	0
7	Was the drug detected in blood (or other fluids) in concentrations known to be toxic?	+1	0	0	0
8	Was the reaction more severe when the dose was increased or less severe when the dose was decreased?	+1	0	0	0
9	Did the patient have a similar reaction to the same or similar drugs in *any* previous exposure?	+1	0	0	0
10	Was the adverse event confirmed by any objective evidence?	+1	0	0	+1
	TOTAL SCORE				+7

The above event was clinically specific; date of drug administration and onset of event was known; thus establishing plausible time relationship. Patient was on oral methyl prednisolone concomitantly but the reaction is most commonly known to occur due to sulfasalazine. Drug was immediately withdrawn on admission suspecting drug hypersensitivity syndrome and treated symptomatically. Patient recovered fully within a week and discharged with methotrexate. Dechallenge in this case is considered positive as patient recovered symptomatically in 7 days after intervention and was discharged with another effective drug .

As Naranjo's algorithm scores to **+7**, the causality falls under category **"Probable"**.

*Using **WHO** scale for this example:*

*(Consider the points in **Bold** while working with WHO scale).*

Patient experienced **reaction** with sulfasalazine and lab data also fluctuated with reasonable **time relationship** of drug intake. The reaction **is less likely** to be attributed to disease and concomitant drug as well. In this case, the suspected drug was **withdrawn** and treated symptomatically following which patient **recovered**. The suspected drug was replaced with another effective drug and patient seemed to be normal. Hence, from the above points we can conclude that the case falls under the category *"Probable"*.

CASE STUDY – 5 [Possible]

A 16 year old ovarian cancer patient had completed 3 cycles of chemotherapy regimen consisting of Inj. Bleomycin, Etoposide and Cisplatin from a Private hospital. Third cycle of chemotherapy was completed on 16/03/15. Later, on 29/03/15 she was brought in Dept of Respiratory Medicine. At the time of admission, she had dyspnea on exertion (severity: grade III), orthopnea, cough with mucoid sputum and intermittent low grade fever.

On chest examination: Bilaterally fine crackle is heard.

Past history: No history of exposure to pets, wheezing, breathlessness and chest pain since childhood.

High resolution computed tomography of thorax suggested bilateral ground glass appearance consistent with Bleomycin toxicity.

Her treating physician diagnosed reaction as *Bleomycin Induced Lung Fibrosis*. Condition of patient further deteriorated during her hospital stay and **expired** after fifteen days.

*Assess **causality for given case using Naranjo's probability scale and explain.***

S. No.	Questions	Yes	No	Don't know	Score
1	Are there previous *conclusive* reports on this reaction?	+1	0	0	+1
2	Did the adverse event appear after the suspected drug was administered?	+2	-1	0	+2
3	Did the adverse reaction improve when the drug was discontinued or a *specific* antagonist was administered?	+1	0	0	0
4	Did the adverse event reappear when the drug was re-administered?	+2	-1	0	0
5	Are there alternative causes (other than the drug) that could on their own have caused the reaction?	-1	+2	0	+2
6	Did the reaction reappear when a placebo was given?	-1	+1	0	0
7	Was the drug detected in blood (or other fluids) in concentrations known to be toxic?	+1	0	0	0

Contd...

S. No.	Questions	Yes	No	Don't know	Score
8	Was the reaction more severe when the dose was increased or less severe when the dose was decreased?	+1	0	0	0
9	Did the patient have a similar reaction to the same or similar drugs in *any* previous exposure?	+1	0	0	0
10	Was the adverse event confirmed by any objective evidence?	+1	0	0	+1
TOTAL SCORE					+7

The **Naranjo scale** score sums to **+7** indicating that the reaction is **probable**. Though there is **plausible time relationship** with drug and reaction, there is no opportunity to see dechallenge as it is a death case. Death cases are always best coded as *"Possible"* if there is **plausible time relationship.** This applies with WHO scale also.

CASE STUDY – 6 [Possible]

A 40 year old male patient, with severe abdominal distension after having food, with complain of hiccups, was prescribed tablet Baclofen 5 mg on 02/2/15. After taking medication, he started vomiting. Patient was not on any other concomitant drug. He is chronic smoker and alcoholic since past 15 years and also a known case of TB. Drug was stopped on 05/2/15. Patient's recovered the next day. No other relevant medical conditions and lab details were mentioned at the time of reporting.

Physician diagnosed the condition as Drug induced *Acute Gastric Enteritis.*

Assess causality for given case using Naranjo's probability scale and explain.

S. No.	Questions	Yes	No	Don't know	Score
1	Are there previous *conclusive* reports on this reaction?	+1	0	0	+1
2	Did the adverse event appear after the suspected drug was administered?	+2	-1	0	+2

Contd...

S. No.	Questions	Yes	No	Don't know	Score
3	Did the adverse reaction improve when the drug was discontinued or a *specific* antagonist was administered?	+1	0	0	+1
4	Did the adverse event reappear when the drug was re-administered?	+2	-1	0	0
5	Are there alternative causes (other than the drug) that could on their own have caused the reaction?	-1	+2	0	-1
6	Did the reaction reappear when a placebo was given?	-1	+1	0	0
7	Was the drug detected in blood (or other fluids) in concentrations known to be toxic?	+1	0	0	0
8	Was the reaction more severe when the dose was increased or less severe when the dose was decreased?	+1	0	0	0
9	Did the patient have a similar reaction to the same or similar drugs in *any* previous exposure?	+1	0	0	0
10	Was the adverse event confirmed by any objective evidence?	+1 [Vomiting in this case]	0	0	+1
	TOTAL SCORE				+4

Using Naranjo's probability scale the above reaction scored +4 which falls under the category **"Possible ADR"**. There is no much detail available for this patient to assess. He is a chronic smoker and alcoholic; and therefore, vomiting is a common symptom of acute gastritis in such patients. Though the patient is a known case of TB, his medications are not known.

One cannot properly assess for any possible association of any drug with the reaction (various conditions are attributed to the cause).

The same explanation applies for **WHO's assessment scale** as well.

CASE STUDY – 7 [Un-assessable]

A 27 year old male patient went to a private physician nearby his locality with complaints of red eyes. The physician prescribed him an eye ointment diagnosing the condition as viral conjunctivitis. After a week the patient came to government hospital having developed fixed drug eruption. He also gave history of intake of medication for headache and ayurvedic drug for persisting knee pain. He had no prescription with him to identify the drugs when he came to hospital following the event.

Assess the causality for the given reaction using Naranjo's Probability Scale and explain.

S. No.	Questions	Yes	No	Don't know	Score
1	Are there previous *conclusive* reports on this reaction?	+1	0	0	0
2	Did the adverse event appear after the suspected drug was administered?	+2	-1	0	0
3	Did the adverse reaction improve when the drug was discontinued or a *specific* antagonist was administered?	+1	0	0	0
4	Did the adverse event reappear when the drug was re-administered?	+2	-1	0	0
5	Are there alternative causes (other than the drug) that could on their own have caused the reaction?	-1	+2	0	0
6	Did the reaction reappear when a placebo was given?	-1	+1	0	0
7	Was the drug detected in blood (or other fluids) in concentrations known to be toxic?	+1	0	0	0
8	Was the reaction more severe when the dose was increased or less severe when the dose was decreased?	+1	0	0	0
9	Did the patient have a similar reaction to the same or similar drugs in *any* previous exposure?	+1	0	0	0
10	Was the adverse event confirmed by any objective evidence?	+1	0	0	0
TOTAL SCORE					0

Sufficient data on drugs used prior to the event is not available. The Patient has got no evidence (prescription) for verification of drugs taken. Hence score is "0" and the relationship is ***"unassessable"***.

[Contributed by Dr. J. Ponni, Pharm.D.]

Appendices (a)

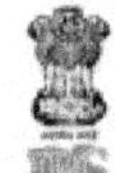

Version-1.3

SUSPECTED ADVERSE DRUG REACTION REPORTING FORM

For VOLUNTARY reporting of Adverse Drug Reaction by Healthcare Professionals

INDIAN PHARMACOPOEIA COMMISSION(National Coordination Centre-Pharmacovigilance Programme of India)

Ministry of Health & Family Welfare, Government of India Sector-23, Raj Nagar, Ghaziabad-201002

A. PATIENT INFORMATION			Reg. No. /IPD No. /OPD No. /CR No. :
1. Patient Initials	2. Age at the time of Event or Date of Birth	3. M ☐ F ☐ Other ☐	AMC Report No. :
		4. Weight__________Kgs	Worldwide Unique No. :

B. SUSPECTED ADVERSE REACTION
5. Event/Reaction start date (dd/mm/yyyy)
6. Event/Reaction stop date (dd/mm/yyyy)
6 (A). Onset Lag Time
7. Describe Event/Reaction with treatment details, if any

12. Relevant tests/ laboratory data with dates

13. Relevant medical/medication history (e.g. allergies, race, pregnancy, smoking, alcohol use, hepatic/renal dysfunction, past surgery etc.)

14. Seriousness of the reaction: No ☐ if Yes ☐(please tick anyone)

☐ Death (__________)   ☐ Congenital-anomaly

☐ Life threatening   ☐ Disability

☐ Hospitalization/Prolonged   ☐ Other Medically important

15. Outcomes

☐ Recovered   ☐ Recovering   ☐ Not recovered

☐ Fatal   ☐ Recovered with sequelae ☐ Unknown

C. SUSPECTED MEDICATION(S)

S.No	8. Name (Brand/Generic)	Manufacturer (if known)	Batch No. / Lot No.	Exp. Date (if known)	Dose used	Route used	Frequency (OD, BD etc.)	Therapy dates Date started	Therapy dates Date stopped	Indication	Causality Assessment
i											
ii											
iii											
iv*											

S.No as per C	9. Action Taken (please tick)							10. Reaction reappeared after reintroduction (please tick)			
	Drug withdrawn	Dose increased	Dose reduced	Dose not changed	Not applicable	Unknown		Yes	No	Effect unknown	Dose (if reintroduced)
i											
ii											
iii											
iv											

11. Concomitant medical product including self-medication and herbal remedies with therapy dates (Exclude those used to treat reaction)

S.No	Name (Brand/Generic)	Dose used	Route used	Frequency (OD, BD, etc.)	Therapy dates Date started	Therapy dates Date stopped	Indication
i							
ii							
iii*							

Additional Information:

D. REPORTER DETAILS
16. Name and Professional Address:__________________
____
Pin:__________E-mail__________________________
Tel. No. (with STD code)______________________
Occupation:__________________Signature:__________
17. Date of this report (dd/mm/yyyy):
Sig. and Name of Receiver-

*use separate page for more information

National Coordination Centre for Pharmacovigilance Programme of India
Ministry of Health & Family Welfare, Government of India
Sector-23, Raj Nagar, Ghaziabad-201002
Tel.: 0120-2783400, 2783401, 2783392, Fax: 0120-2783311
www.ipc.nic.in

ADVICE ABOUT REPORTING

A. What to report?

➤ Report serious adverse drug reactions. A reaction is serious when the patient outcome is:
  - Death
  - Life-threatening
  - Hospitalization (initial or prolonged)
  - Disability (significant, persistent or permanent)
  - Congenital anomaly
  - Required intervention to prevent permanent impairment or damage

➤ Report non-serious, known or unknown, frequent or rare adverse drug reactions due to Medicines, Vaccines and Herbal products etc.

  Note- Adverse Event Following Immunization can also be reported in Serious AEFI case Notification Form available on http://www.ipc.gov.in)

B. Who can report?

➤ All healthcare professionals (Clinicians, Dentists, Pharmacists and Nurses etc) can report adverse drug reactions

C. Where to report?

➤ Duly filled inSuspected Adverse Drug Reaction Reporting Form can be sent to the nearest Adverse Drug Reaction Monitoring Centre (AMC) or directly to the National Coordination Centre (NCC) for PvPI.

➤ Call on Helpline (Toll Free) 1800 180 3024 to report ADRs or directly mail this filled form to pvpi@ipcindia.net or pvpi.ipcindia@gmail.com

➤ A list of nationwide AMCs is available at:
  http://www.ipc.gov.in, http://www.ipc.gov.in/PvPI/pv_home.html

D. What happens to the submitted information?

➤ Information provided in this form is handled in strict confidence. The causality assessment is carried out at AMCs by using WHO-UMC scale. The analyzed forms are forwarded to the NCC through ADR database. Finally the data is analyzed and forwarded to the Global Pharmacovigilance Database managed by WHO Uppsala Monitoring Centre in Sweden.

➤ The reports are periodically reviewed by the NCC-PvPI. The information generated on the basis of these reports helps in continuous assessment of the benefit-risk ratio of medicines.

➤ The Signal Review Panel of PvPI to review the data and suggest any interventions that may be required.

E. Mandatory fields for suspected ADR reporting form

➤ Patient initials, age at onset of reaction, reaction term(s), date of onset of reaction, suspected medication(s) and reporter information.

For ADRs Reporting

➤ **E-mail:**pvpi@ipcindia.net **or** pvpi.ipcindia@gmail.com
➤ *PvPI Helpline (Toll Free):*1800 180 3024*(9:00 AM to 5:30 PM, Monday-Friday)*
➤ *ADR Mobile App: "ADR PvPI"*

Guidance for Filling up the ADR Form

A. Patient Information

1. ***Patient initials:*** A reporter should only mention the initials of a patient instead of the full name. For e.g.: Madhu Gupta should be written as MG.

2. ***Age at time of event or date of birth:*** A reporter must report either the date of birth or age of the patient at the time the event or reaction occurred.

3. ***Sex:*** A reporter must mention the gender of the patient.

4. ***Weight:*** The weight of the patient should be in kilograms.

B. Suspected Adverse Reaction

5. ***Date of reaction started:*** A reporter must report the date on which the reaction was first observed.

6. ***Date of recovery:*** If the reaction recovered, the date on which the reaction recovered should be reported.

7. ***Describe reaction:*** A reporter must briefly describe the event in terms of nature, localization etc. For example patient developed erythematous maculopapular rash over upper and lower limbs.

C. Suspected Medications

8. The details of suspected medication(s) such as the *drug name (brand or generic name), manufacturer, batch no/lot no, expiry date, dose used, route used, frequency, dates of therapy started and stopped, and indication of use* must be provided by the reporter.

9. ***De-challenge details:*** A reporter must report the status of de-challenge as:

   - 'Yes' - if reaction abated or reduced after de-challenge

   - 'No' - if reaction did not abated after de-challenge

   - 'Unknown' - if information on de-challenge is not confirmed or not known

- **'Not Applicable' or 'NA'** - if de-challenge is not possible as in case of anaphylaxis, life threatening events, anaesthetic drugs or where a single dose is given.
- **'Reduced dose'** - If dose at which the reaction occurred is reduced

Note: Also mention the reduced dose

10. *Re-challenge details:* A reporter must report the status of re-challenge as:

    - **'Yes'** - if reaction reappeared after re-challenge
    - **'No'** - if reaction did not reappear after re-challenge
    - **'Unknown'** - if information on re-challenge is not confirmed or not known
    - **'Not Applicable' or 'NA'** - if re-challenge is not applicable as in the case of injections.
    - **'Re-introduced dose'**- If the drug is reintroduced is it a reduced dose or is it the same dose at which adverse event occurred initially.

11. *Concomitant drugs:* A reporter should include all the details of concomitant drugs including self medication, OTC medication, herbal remedies with therapy dates (start and stop date.)

12. *Relevant tests/ laboratory data:* A reporter must mention any laboratory data (if available) relevant to the adverse event that occurred.

13. *Other relevant history:* A reporter must mention any relevant history pertaining to the patient including pre-existing medical conditions (e.g. allergies, pregnancy, smoking, alcohol use, hepatic/renal dysfunction).

14. *Seriousness of the reaction:* If any event is serious in nature, a reporter must select the appropriate reason for seriousness:

    - **'Death'** - if the patient died due to the adverse event
    - **'Life-threatening'** - if patient was at substantial risk of dying because of the adverse event
    - **'Hospitalisation/prolonged'** - if the adverse event led to hospitalization or increased the hospital stay of the patient

- **'Disability'** - if the adverse event resulted in a substantial disruption of a person's ability to conduct normal life functions

- **'Congenital anomaly'** - if exposure of drug prior to conception or during pregnancy may have resulted in an adverse outcome in the child.

- **'Required intervention to prevent permanent impairment/damage'** - if medical or surgical intervention was necessary to preclude permanent impairment of a body function, or prevent permanent damage to a body structure

- **'Other'** - when the event does not fit the other outcomes, but the event may put the patient at risk and may require medical or surgical intervention to prevent one of the other outcomes. Examples include serious blood dyscrasias (blood disorders) or seizures/convulsions that do not result in hospitalization, development of drug dependence or drug abuse

15. *Outcomes:* The reporter must tick the outcome of the event as:

    - **'Fatal'** - if the patient dies due to the adverse event

    - **'Continuing'** - if the patient is continuing to have the symptoms of the adverse event which occurred

    - **'Recovering'** - if the patient is recovering from the existing adverse event

    - **'Recovered'** - if the patient has recovered from the event

    - **'Unknown'** - if the outcome is not known

D. Reporter

16. *Name and Professional address:* A reporter must mention his/her name and professional address on the form. The identity of the reporter will be maintained confidential

17. *Causality assessment:* The reporter (if trained) must perform the causality assessment.

18. *Date of report:* Mention the date on which he/she reported the adverse event.

Note: For quality reporting of ICSRs all the above mentioned fields are essential. In case of incomplete information, the reporter must take care that at least mandatory fields are present. Following are the mandatory fields for a valid case report:

- *Patient information:* initials, age at onset of reaction, gender.
- *Suspected adverse reaction:* A reaction term(s), date of onset of reaction.
- *Suspected medication:* Drug(s) name, dose, date of therapy started, indication of use, seriousness, outcome, de-challenge and re-challenge details.
- *Reporter:* Name and address, causality assessment, date of report.

Appendices (c)

Version 1.0
संस्करण 1.0

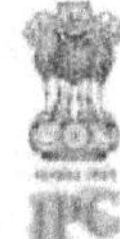

MEDICINES SIDE EFFECT REPORTING FORM (FOR CONSUMERS)
औषधि दुष्प्रभाव सूचना फॉर्म (उपभोक्ताओं के लिए)

Indian Pharmacopoeia Commission, National Coordination Centre - Pharmacovigilance Programme of India, Ministry of Health & Family Welfare, Government of India.

भारतीय भेषज संहिता आयोग, राष्ट्रीय समन्वय केंद्र — भारतीय फार्माकोविजिलेंस कार्यक्रम, स्वास्थ्य एवं परिवार कल्याण मंत्रालय, भारत सरकार।

1.Patient Details/ रोगी का विवरण

Patient Initials/ रोगी के आद्याक्षर: ☐☐   Gender/ लिंग (v): Male/ पुरूष ☐ Female/ स्त्री ☐ Other/ अन्य ☐   Age (Year or Month)/ आयु (वर्ष या माह) :

2. Health Information/ स्वास्थ्य संबंधी जानकारी

a. Reason(s) for taking medicine(s)(Disease/Symptoms)/ दवा(दवाएं) लेने का कारण (रोग / लक्षण):

b. Medicines Advised by/ दवाई की सलाह देने वाला (v): Doctor/ डॉक्टर ☐ Pharmacist/ फार्मासिस्ट ☐ Friends/Relatives/ मित्र / रिश्तेदार ☐
Self (Past disease experienced/No past disease experienced)/ स्वयं (पूर्व बीमारी का अनुभव / पूर्व बीमारी का कोई अनुभव नहीं) ☐

3. Details of Person Reporting the Side Effect/ दुष्प्रभाव की सूचना देने वाले व्यक्ति का विवरण

Name (Optional)/ नाम (वैकल्पिक):

Address/ पता:

Telephone No/ टेलीफोन नं:   Email/ ईमेल:

4. Details of Medicine Taking/Taken/ ली जा रही है / ली जा चुकी दवाई का विवरण

Name of Medicines/ दवाइयों के नाम	Quantity of Medicines taken (e.g. 250 mg, Two times a day)/ ली गई दवाई की मात्रा (उदाहरण के लिए 250 मिग्रा, एक दिन में दो बार)	Expiry Date of Medicines/ दवा के निष्क्रिय होने की तिथि	Date of Start of Medicines/ दवाइया आरंभ करने की तिथि	Date of Stop of Medicines/ दवाइयां रोकने की तिथि

Dosage form/खुराक का स्वरूप (v) : Tablet/ गोली (टेबलेट) ☐ Capsule/ कैप्सूल ☐ Injection/ इंजेक्शन ☐ Oral Liquids/ मौखिक तरल ☐ If Others (Please Specify................../यदि अन्य (कृपया निर्दिष्ट करें............)

5. About the Side Effect/ दुष्प्रभाव के बारे में

When did the side effect start?/ दुष्प्रभाव की शुरूआत कब हुई थी? [ ]   Side Effect is still Continuing (Yes/No)/

When did the side effect stop?/ दुष्प्रभाव कब समाप्त हुआ था? [ ]   क्या दुष्प्रभाव जारी है (हां / नहीं) [ ]

6.How bad was the Side Effect? (Please v the boxes that Apply)/ दुष्प्रभाव कितने हानिकारक थे? (कृपया जो लागू हो, उस पर √ का निशान लगाएं)

☐ Did not affect daily activities/ दैनिक गतिविधियां प्रभावित नहीं हुई थी   ☐ Affect daily activities/ दैनिक गतिविधियां प्रभावित हुईं
☐ Admitted to hospital/ अस्पताल ले जाना पड़ा   ☐ Death/ मृत्यु
☐ Others/ अन्य

7.Describe the Side Effect (What did you do to manage the side effect?)/ दुष्प्रभाव की व्याख्या करें (आपने दुष्प्रभावों से छुटकारा प्राप्त करने के लिए क्या किया)?

Please turn the page to read the instructions
निर्देशों को पढ़ने के लिए कृपया पेज पलटें

Instructions to Complete the Reporting Form
सूचना फॉर्म को पूरा करने के लिए निर्देश

Section 1 - Patient Details	**निर्देश 1 – रोगी का विवरण**

Section 1 - Patient Details

- In patient initial, write first letter of the name and first letter of the surname (e.g. Pradeep Sharma-PS).
- Provide personal information (Gender, Age).

Section -2 Health Information

- Provide reason(s) for taking medicines and medicines advised by (Doctor, Pharmacists, Friends/ Relatives and Self).

Section 3 - Details of Person Reporting the Side Effect

- Provide the name (optional), address; telephone no. and email are necessary to assess the report.

Section 4 - Details of the Medicines Taking/Taken

- Give all details about the Medicines (Name of Medicines, Quantity of Medicines taken, Expiry Date, start and stop date of Medicines) that have caused side effect.
- Please provide Dosage form (Tablets, Capsule, injections, Oral liquid) and if others please specify.

Section 5 - About the Side Effect

- Provide side effect start and stop dates and also specify whether the side effect is still continuing.

Section 6 - How bad was the Side Effect

- Please tick marks the appropriate boxes that apply.

Section 7- Describe the Side Effect

- Please describe the details of side effect and what treatment was taken to manage the side effect.

निर्देश 1 – रोगी का विवरण

- रोगी के आद्याक्षर में, नाम का पहला अक्षर लिखे और उपनाम का प्रथम अक्षर लिखे (जैसे प्रदीप शर्मा–प्रश)।
- व्यक्तिगत जानकारी (लिंग, आयु) प्रदान करें।

निर्देश –2 स्वास्थ्य संबंधी जानकारी

- दवा लेने के कारण और परामर्शदाता का नाम दे (डॉक्टर, फार्मासिस्ट, मित्र/रिश्तेदार और स्वयं)।

निर्देश 3 – दुष्प्रभाव की रिपोर्ट करने वाले व्यक्ति का विवरण दें

- रिपोर्ट के मूल्यांकन हेतु नाम (विकल्पिक), पता, टेलीफोन नं और ई–मेल उपलब्ध कराएं।

निर्देश 4 – ली जा रही है / ली जा चुकी दवाइयों का विवरण

- उन दवाइयों (दवाइयों का नाम, ली गई दवाइयां, निष्क्रिय होने की तिथि, दवाइया शुरू करने एवं रोकने की तिथि) का विवरण दें जिनके कारण आपको दुष्प्रभाव हुआ है।
- खुराक का स्वरूप (गोली (टेबलेट), कैप्सूल, इजेक्शन, मौखिक तरल (पीने वाली दवा) और यदि कोई अन्य हो तो निर्दिष्ट करें।

निर्देश 5 – दुष्प्रभाव के प्रभाव के बारे में

- दुष्प्रभाव आरंभ और समाप्त होने की तिथि बताएं और यह भी निर्दिष्ट करें कि क्या दुष्प्रभाव अभी भी जारी है।

निर्देश 6 – दुष्प्रभाव कितने हानिकारक थे?

- कृपया उचित डब्बे पर निशान लगाएं।

निर्देश 7– दुष्प्रभाव की व्याख्या करें

- कृपया दुष्प्रभाव का विवरण और उस दुष्प्रभाव से छुटकारा पाने के लिए क्या उपचार किया गया, विवेचना करें।

इस फॉर्म को पूरा करने के लिए अपना समय देने हेतु आपका धन्यवाद।

Appendices (d)

Serious AEFI Case Notification Form – ADR Monitoring Center*

ICSR No. ___________________   **Reporting Format No.**

Name & address of ADR Monitoring center (AMC):

Patient Name

Age: _________   Sex: Male/Female

Father/Husband's Name

Complete Address of the Case with landmarks *(Street name, house number, village, block, Tehsil, PIN No., Telephone No. etc.)*

P I N -   P H O N E -

Date of Vaccination: ___ / ___ / ___

Address of health facility where vaccinated (include name of village/urban area, block, DISTRICT and STATE)#:

Name of vaccines with dose received (if known)													
Date of first symptom	D	D	M	M	Y	Y	Y	Y	Time of first symptom	H	H	M	M	(AM/PM)
Hospitalization:(No/ Yes) Date-	D	D	M	M	Y	Y	Y	Y	Time of hospitalization	H	H	M	M	(AM/PM)

Name and address of hospital (if hospitalized):   CR No./MRD No _________________

Current status (encircle)	Death / Still Hospitalized / Recovered & Discharged with sequelae /Recovered completely and discharged / Left Against Medical Advice (LAMA) / Not hospitalized

If died, Date of Death	D	D	M	M	Y	Y	Y	Y	Time of Death	H	H	M	M	(AM/PM)

Describe AEFI (signs and symptoms):

Name & signature of AMC Coordinator/ Medical officer:

Email:

Contact No.

*Date form sent to District Immunization Officer# **(where patient was vaccinated)**- ___ / ___ / ___

*Date form sent to State Immunization Officer# **(where patient was vaccinated)**- ___ / ___ / ___

*Date form sent to PVPI, Ghaziabad- ___ / ___ / ___

*Date form sent to Immunization Division / AEFI Secretariat (aefiindia@gmail.com)- ___ / ___ / ___

Name & signature of Pharmacovigilance Associate:

E mail:

Contact number:

#The case is to be notified to the DIO of the district where the vaccine was administered.
*This form should be scanned and emailed simultaneously to DIO, SEPIO, PVPI and AEFI Secretariat

Appendix (e)

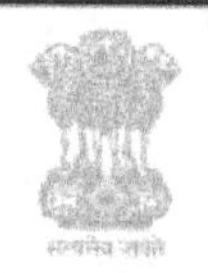 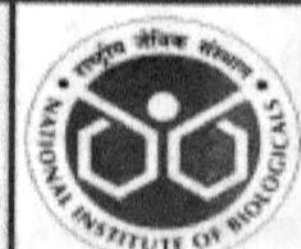

National Institute of Biologicals
Ministry of Health & Family Welfare, Govt. of India
(National Coordinating Center)
HAEMOVIGILANCE PROGRAMME OF INDIA

Transfusion Reaction Reporting Form (TRRF) For Blood & Blood Components & Plasma Products

* Mandatory Field

(A) Patient Information

Hospital Code No.:

| Patient Initials*: | | Gender*: | | | Blood Group*: | |

| Hospital Admission No.*: | | Age/Date of Birth*: | | ......Yrs | ......Month | ....Days | .... Hrs | ...... Mins |

Primary Diagnosis*:

Medical History:

(B) Transfusion Reaction Details*

Was the patient under anaesthesia during transfusion: Yes/No   if Yes type : GA/Spinal/LA

| Pre-transfusion Vitals: | Temp: | Pulse: | BP: | RR: | SPO2: |
| Vitals at the time of reaction: | Temp: | Pulse: | BP: | RR: | SPO2: |

Please tick mark the relevant signs and symptoms listed below

Generalised			Pain		Respiratory		Renal		Circulatory	
☐ Fever	☐ Anxiety		☐ Chest Pain		☐ Dyspnoea		☐ Haematuria		☐ Tachycardia	
☐ Chills	☐ Itching (Pruritus)		☐ Abdominal		☐ Wheeze		☐ Haemoglobinuria		☐ Hypertension	
☐ Rigors	☐ Edema (Site)		☐ Back/Flank Pain		☐ Cough		☐ Oliguria		☐ Hypotension	
☐ Nausea	☐ Juandice		☐ Infusion Site Pain		☐ Hypoxemia		☐ Other		☐ Raised JVP	
☐ Urticaria	☐ Other		☐ Other		☐				☐ Arrhythmias	
☐ Flushing					Bilateral Infiltrates on				☐ Other	
☐ Restlessness					Chest X-ray					
☐ Vomiting					☐ Other					

Any Other(Specify) : ....

(C) Transfusion Product(s) Details*

Select*	Select Component	Select Indication	Date & Time of Issue of Blood Component	Date & Time of onset Transfusion	Unit Id (Transfused)	Blood Group	Volume Transfused (ml)	Expiry date of Blood Component	Manufacturer of Blood Bag	Batch / Lot No. of the Blood Bag	1st time/ repeat Transfusion
☐	Whole blood										
☐	Packed Red blood cells (PRBC)										☐ 1st Time
☐	Buffy coat depleted PRBC										
☐	Leucofiltered PRBC										
☐	Random Donor platelets/ pooled										☐ Repeat 1 to 10
☐	Apheresis Platelets										
☐	Fresh Frozen Plasma										
☐	Cryoprecipitate										☐ Repeat > 10
☐	Any Other										

Add New Plasma Product

Select	Plasma Product	Indication	Date of Administration	Manufacturer	Expiry Date of the Plasma Product	Batch No. / Lot No.	1st Time / Repeat
							☐ 1st Time ☐ Repeat 1 to 10 ☐ Repeat > 10

(D) Investigations

☐ Clerical Checks Specify Error Found if any: ______________

Investigation	Pre-transfusion sample			Post-transfusion sample		
☐ Repeat Blood Grouping	O+ /A+ /B+ /AB+ /O- /A- /B- /AB-			O+ /A+ /B+ /AB+ /O- /A- /B- /AB-		
☐ Repeat Crossmatch	☐ Compatible	☐ InCompatible	☐ Not Done	☐ Compatible	☐ InCompatible	☐ Not Done
☐ Repeat Antibody screen	☐ Negative	☐ Positive	☐ Not Done	☐ Negative	☐ Positive	☐ Not Done
☐ Antibody Identification						
☐ Direct antiglobulin test	☐ Negative	☐ Positive	☐ Not Done	☐ Negative	☐ Positive	☐ Not Done
☐ Hemoglobin						
☐ Plasma Hemoglobin						
☐ Urine hemoglobin						
☐ Bilirubin (Total/conjugated)						
☐ Platelet count						
☐ PT/INR						
☐ Blood culture of Blood Bag	☐ Negative	☐ Positive	☐ Not Done	Specify Organism if positive ______		
☐ Blood culture of Patient	☐ Negative	☐ Positive	☐ Not Done	☐ Negative	☐ Positive	☐ Not Done
	Specify Organism if positive ______			Specify Organism if positive ______		

☐ Chest X-ray of the patient in case of suspected TRALI

In case of Non-immune hemolysis (which of the following was the case?)

☐ Hemolysis due to freezing of PRBC Units
☐ Hemolysis due to inappropriate warming of PRBC Units
☐ Hemolysis due to infusion of any other fluid through same BT set. Specify Fluid: ______________
☐ Mechanical damage

In Case of ABO Mismatch (which of the following was the case?)

☐ Wrong Blood in tube
☐ Grouping error
☐ Labelling error
☐ Wrong unit transfused

(E) Nature of Adverse Reaction(s)*

Select	Reaction	Date & Time of Onset of Reaction	Date & Time of Recovery	Outcome
☐	Febrile Non Haemolytic Reactions (FNHTR) 1° C rise in temperature ☐ 2° C rise in temperature ☐ Only Chills & Rigors ☐			☐ 1. Death following the Adverse Reaction(s)
☐	Allergic reaction			
☐	Anaphylaxis			
☐	Immunological Haemolysis due to ABO Incompatibility			
☐	Immunological Haemolysis due to other Allo-Antibodies			
☐	Non Immunological Haemolysis			☐ 2. Recovered
☐	Hypotensive Transfusion Reaction			
☐	Transfusion Related Acute Lung Injury (TRALI) Definite ☐ Possible ☐			
☐	Transfusion Associated Dyspnoea (TAD)			
☐	Transfusion Associated Circulatory Overload (TACO)			☐
☐	Transfusion Transmitted Bacterial Infection			3. Recovered with Sequelae
☐	Transfusion Transmitted Parasitic Infection (Malaria)			
☐	Post Transfusion Purpura			
☐	Transfusion Associated Graft versus Host Disease (TAGvHD)			☐ 4. Unknown
☐	Other Reaction (s) ______________ Add New ______________			

(F) Imputability Assessment*

S. No.	Reaction Term	Transfusion Product/ Component	*Imputability Assessment (Please mention from the below list)

*Imputability: 1. Definite (Certain), 2. Probable (Likely), 3. Possible, 4. Unlikely (Doubtful), 5. Excluded, 6. Not Assessed

Monthly Denominator Reporting Form

Hospital Code : ______________   Month/Year: ______________

Blood Component	No. of Units Issued
1) Fresh Frozen Plasma	
2) Whole Blood	
3) Packed Red Blood Cells (PRBC)	
4) Buffy Coat Depleted PRBC	
5) Leucofiltered PRBC	
6) Random Donor Platelets/ Pooled	
7) Apheresis Platelets	
8) Cryoprecipitate	
9) Any Other ______	

Appendix (f)

BLOOD DONOR ADVERSE REACTION REPORTING FORM

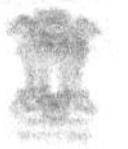

National Institute of Biologicals
Ministry of Health & Family Welfare, Govt. of India
NATIONAL BLOOD DONOR VIGILANCE PROGRAMME
(Haemovigilance Programme of India)
Blood Donor Adverse Reaction Reporting Form

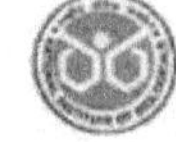

I) Donor Information

Donor Id _____________________   Type of Donation _____________
Sex _____________   Donor Type _____________
Weight of Donor (KG) _______________   Venipuncture _____________
Age/Date of Birth _______________

II) Details of Blood Collected

Lot No.of Blood Bag _______________   Volume of Blood Collected (ml) _____________

Manufacturer of Blood Bag _____________   Expiry Date of Blood Bag _____________

III) Type of Complications

A1-Complications mainly characterized by the occurrence of blood outside the vessels
   (a)   Haematoma (bruise)
   (b)   Arterial puncture
   (c)   Delayed(bleeding/Re-bleeding)

A2-Complications mainly characterized by pain
   (a)   Nerve injury/irritation
   (b)   Other Painful arm

A3-Localised infection/inflammation along the course of a vein
   (a)   Deep venous thrombosis (DVT)
   (b)   Arteriovenous fistula
   (c)   Compartment syndrome
   (d)   Brachial artery pseudoaneurysm

B-Complications mainly with generalized symptoms: Vasovagal reactions
   (a)   LOC < 60 sec
   (b)   LOC > 60 sec
   (c)   With injury
   (d)   Without injury
   (e)   Within Blood collection facility
   (f)   Outside blood collection facility

C-Complications related to apheresis
   (a)   Citrate reaction
   (b)   Haemolysis
   (c)   Air embolism
   (d)   Infiltration of IV fluids

D-Allergic reactions
   (a)   Allergy (local)
   (b)   Generalised allergic reaction (anaphylactic reaction)

E-Other serious complications related to blood donation
   (a)   Acute cardiac symptoms
   (b)   Myocardial infarction(MI)
   (c)   Cardiac arrest
   (d)   Death

IV) Outcomes

☐ Resolved
☐ On Follow Up
☐ Recovered with Sequelae
☐ Permanently Disabled
☐ Death following the Adverse Reactions

V) Imputability

☐ Definite (Certain)
☐ Probable (Likely)
☐ Possible
☐ Unlikely (Doubtful)
☐ Excluded

VI) Reporter _____________

Date of Report _______________

(D) Investigations

☐ Clerical Checks — Specify Error Found if any:

Investigation	Pre-transfusion sample	Post-transfusion sample
* ☐ Repeat Blood Grouping	O+ /A+ /B+ /AB+ /O- /A- /B- /AB-	O+ /A+ /B+ /AB+ /O- /A- /B- /AB-
* ☐ Repeat Crossmatch	☐ Compatible ☐ InCompatible ☐ Not Done	☐ Compatible ☐ InCompatible ☐ Not Done
* ☐ Repeat Antibody screen	☐ Negative ☐ Positive ☐ Not Done	☐ Negative ☐ Positive ☐ Not Done
☐ Antibody Identification		
* ☐ Direct antiglobulin test	☐ Negative ☐ Positive ☐ Not Done	☐ Negative ☐ Positive ☐ Not Done
☐ Hemoglobin		
☐ Plasma Hemoglobin		
☐ Urine hemoglobin		
☐ Bilirubin (Total/conjugated)		
☐ Platelet count		
☐ PT/INR		
* ☐ Blood culture of Blood Bag	☐ Negative ☐ Positive ☐ Not Done Specify Organism if positive	
* ☐ Blood culture of Patient	☐ Negative ☐ Positive ☐ Not Done Specify Organism if positive	☐ Negative ☐ Positive ☐ Not Done Specify Organism if positive
☐ Chest X-ray of the patient in case of suspected TRALI		

In case of Non-immune hemolysis (which of the following was the case?)

☐ Hemolysis due to freezing of PRBC Units
☐ Hemolysis due to inappropriate warming of PRBC Units
☐ Hemolysis due to infusion of any other fluid through same BT set. Specify Fluid:
☐ Mechanical damage

In Case of ABO Mismatch (which of the following was the case?)

☐ Wrong Blood in tube
☐ Grouping error
☐ Labelling error
☐ Wrong unit transfused

(E) Nature of Adverse Reaction(s)*

Select	Reaction	Date & Time of Onset of Reaction	Date & Time of Recovery	Outcome
☐	Febrile Non Haemolytic Reactions (FNHTR) 1° C rise in temperature ☐ 2° C rise in temperature ☐ Only Chills & Rigors ☐			☐ 1. Death following the Adverse Reaction(s)
☐	Allergic reaction			
☐	Anaphylaxis			
☐	Immunological Haemolysis due to ABO Incompatibility			
☐	Immunological Haemolysis due to other Allo-Antibodies			
☐	Non Immunological Haemolysis			☐ 2. Recovered
☐	Hypotensive Transfusion Reaction			
☐	Transfusion Related Acute Lung Injury (TRALI) Definite ☐ Possible ☐			
☐	Transfusion Associated Dyspnoea (TAD)			
☐	Transfusion Associated Circulatory Overload (TACO)			☐ 3. Recovered with Sequelae
☐	Transfusion Transmitted Bacterial Infection			
☐	Transfusion Transmitted Parasitic Infection (Malaria)			
☐	Post Transfusion Purpura			
☐	Transfusion Associated Graft versus Host Disease (TAGvHD)			☐ 4. Unknown
☐	Other Reaction (s) Add New			

(F) Imputability Assessment*

S. No.	Reaction Term	Transfusion Product/ Component	*Imputability Assessment (Please mention from the below list)

*Imputability: 1. Definite (Certain), 2. Probable (Likely), 3. Possible, 4. Unlikely (Doubtful), 5. Excluded, 6. Not Assessed

Monthly Denominator Reporting Form *

Hospital Code : Month/Year:

Blood Component	No.of Units Issued
1) Fresh Frozen Plasma	
2) Whole Blood	
3) Packed Red Blood Cells (PRBC)	
4) Buffy Coat Depleted PRBC	
5) Leucofiltered PRBC	
6) Random Donor Platelets/ Pooled	
7) Apheresis Platelets	
8) Cryoprecipitate	
9) Any Other_______	

Appendix (g)

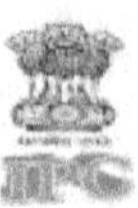

MEDICAL DEVICE ADVERSE EVENT REPORTING FORM

Materiovigilance Programme of India (MvPI)

This form is intended to collect information on Medical Devices Adverse Event in India. The form is designed to be used voluntarily by Manufacturer/Importer/Distributor of Medical Devices, Healthcare Professionals and anyone with direct/indirect knowledge of Medical Devices Adverse Event.

General Information

1. Date of Report :
2. Type of Report : Initial ☐   Follow up ☐   Final ☐   Trend ☐
3. Reporter Reference for MDMC only: • Centre   • Location   • Month-Year   • Case No.

Reporter Details

1. Type of Reporter : (a) Manufacturer ☐   (b) Importer ☐   (c) Distributor ☐   (d) Healthcare Professional ☐

     (e) Patient ☐   (f) Others ☐ **specify**

2. In case, where the reporter is not manufacturer, fill the following details:-

   (a) Has the reporter informed the incident to the manufacturer?

        Yes ☐   No ☐

   (b) Is the reporter also submitting the report on behalf of the manufacturer?

        Yes ☐   No ☐

3. Reporter contact information:

   a) Name   :
   b) Address   :
   c) Tel. /Mobile :
   d) Email   :

Device Category

Medical Device	In Vitro Diagnostics (IVD)	Medical Equipments / Machines

I. Therapeutic ☐ Diagnostic ☐
    Both ☐ Preventive ☐
    Assistive ☐
	I. Kits ☐	I. Therapeutic ☐ Diagnostic ☐

	II. Reagents ☐	II. Therapeutic & Diagnostic ☐
	III. Calibrator ☐	III. Preventive ☐
II. Implantable device ☐	IV. Control Material ☐	IV. Assistive ☐
Non-Implantable device ☐	V. Others ☐	V. Imaging ☐
III. Invasive ☐ Non-Invasive ☐	VI. IVD electronic reader/ ☐	VI. Invasive ☐ Non-Invasive ☐
IV. Single use device ☐	Analyzer	VII. Others ☐
Reusable device ☐		
Reuse of manufacture marked Single use device ☐		
V. Sterile ☐ Non Sterile ☐		
VI. Personal use / Homecare use ☐		

Instruction for use Section A-F

- *If Medical Devices/Equipments/Machines : Please fill all the sections i.e. A, B, C, D, E & F*
- *If in Vitro Diagnostics (IVD) : Please fill sections i.e. A (except 6, 7, 8, 13, 14 & 16), B (except 1, 2, 6 & 8), D, E, & F*

Device Name / Trade Name / Brand Name:

Details	Name	Address
Manufacturer		
Importer		
Distributor		

1. a) Is the device notified/regulated in India : Yes ☐ No ☐

   b) Device Risk Classification as per India MDR 2017 : A ☐ B ☐ C ☐ D ☐

2. License No. (Manufacture/Import) :

3. Catalogue No. :

4. Model No. :

5. Lot / Batch No. :

6. Serial No. :

7. Software Version :

8. Associated Devices / Accessories :

9. Nomenclature Code if applicable; GMDN/UMDNS :

10. UDI No. (If applicable) :

11. Installation Date :

12. Expiration Date :

13. Last preventive maintenance date (dd/mm/yyyy) :

14. Last calibration date (dd/mm/yyyy) :

15. Year of manufacturing :

16. How long was device/Equipment/Machine in use :

17. Availability of device for evaluation : Yes ☐ No ☐

    If no, was the device destroyed ☐ Still in use ☐ return to manufacturer or importer/distributor ☐

18. Is the usage of device as per manufacturer claim /Instruction for use/user manual: Yes ☐ No ☐

    If no specify usage

19. For devices not regulated / notified in India : Regulator / Regulatory status in country of origin

1. Date of Event / Near miss incident:
2. Date of Implant/Explant (If applicable):
3. Location of Event:

   Hospital Premise ☐ Manufacture/Distributor premise ☐

   Home ☐ Others ☐
4. Device Operator:-

   Healthcare Professional ☐ Patient ☐ Others ☐

   Problem noted prior to use/near miss event ☐
5. Device disposition / Current location:

   a) Returned to company ☐ If yes, date ....../....../........

   b) Remains implanted in patient ☐

   c) Within the healthcare facility ☐

   d) At patient home ☐

   e) Destroyed ☐

   f) Others (specify) ☐
6. Is device in use after incidence : Yes ☐ No ☐

7. Serious event: ☐

   If serious, Tick the appropriate reason

   a) Death (DD/MM/YY) ☐ ..../............/............

   b) Life Threatening ☐

   c) Disability or permanent damage ☐

   d) Hospitalization ☐

   e) Congenital anomaly /birth defect ☐

   f) Any other serious (Imp. medical event) ☐

   g) Required intervention to prevent / permanent ☐
      Impairment / damage device
8. Non serious event ☐
9. Whether other medical devices were used at same time
   with above device if yes, please specify name(s)/use(s)

10. Detail description of Event:-

For manufacturer/authorized representative use only

11. Frequency of occurrence of similar Adverse Event in India in past 3 years	Year	No. of Similar Adverse Events	Total No. Supplied	Frequency of Occurrence (%)
12. Frequency of occurrence of similar Adverse Event in globally in past 3 years	Year	No. of Similar Adverse Events	Total No. Supplied	Frequency of Occurrence (%)

1. Patient Hospital ID :
2. Patient Initial :
3. Age :
4. Gender : Male ☐ Female ☐ Others ☐
5. Weight :
6. Other relevant history, including pre-existing medical conditions

7. Patient Outcomes:

   a) Recovered Date (DD/MM/YY) ☐ ....../....../......

   b) Not yet recovered ☐

   c) Death (DD/MM/YY) ☐ ....../....../......

   d) Others ☐

      Please specify

1. Name   :
2. Address   :
3. Contact Person Name at the site of event   :
4. Tel. No.   :

(E) Causality Assessment

1. Investigation action taken:

2. Root cause of problem (Applicable for follow up / final reports):

(F) Manufacturer/Authorized Representative Investigation & Action taken

1. Manufacturer/Authorized Representative device risk analysis report:

2. Corrective / preventive action taken:

3. Device history review:

10. Detail description of Event:-

1. Investigation action taken:

2. Root cause of problem (Applicable for follow up / final reports):

1. Manufacturer/Authorized Representative device risk analysis report:

2. Corrective / preventive action taken:

3. Device history review:

Where to report?

Duly filled **Medical Device Adverse Event Reporting Form** can be sent to Indian Pharmacopoeia Commission, Ministry of Health and Family Welfare, Government of India, Sector-23, Rajnagar, Ghaziabad-20002, Tel-0120-2783400, 2783401 and 2783392, FAX:0120-2783311 or email to mvpi.ipcindia@gmail.com Or Call on Helpline no. 1800 180 3024 to report Adverse event.

Partnering Organizations

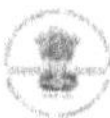 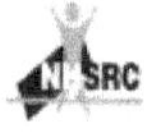 

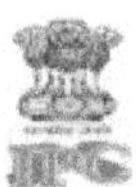

FIELD SAFETY CORRECTIVE ACTION NOTIFICATION (FSCA) FORM

1. Before filling this form, the reporter collects and collates the prescribed information in the form.
2. This form will serve as the reporting tool in lieu with the Medical Devices Rules, 2017.
   Fourth Schedule
   [See rule 20(2), 21(2), 34(2), 63(1) and 64(1)] Part II (ii) (b) and Appendix II for intimating, notifying CDSCO for any Field Safety Corrective Action (FSCA) in relation to medical device product recall and other corrective action.
3. A scanned signed copy of PDF version of this form is to be sent to CDSCO via email to dci.nic.in
4. Additional information that may be pertinent for the completion of this form can be provided as an attachment.
5. All the field safety notices will be published on the CDSCO website and the reporter holds the full responsibility for the information contained in the Field Safety Notification and reporter must indemnify CDSCO for all losses, claims, demands, liabilities, causes of action, expenses of any kind arising from CDSCO's publication of the FSN.

Primary Information

1.	Type of Field Safety Corrective Action (FSCA)	☐ Product Recall
		☐ Other Corrective actions
2.	Type of Report	☐ Notification
		☐ Preliminary Report
		☐ Final Report
3.	Date of Report (dd/mm/yy)	
4.	Reference Number (auto generated by system)	

Particulars of Reporters

1.	Contact Person Name	
2.	Job Title	
3.	Telephone Numbers	
4.	Email Address	
5.	Office Address	
6.	Local Contact Details (if reporter not based in India)	

1.	Device Name	
2.	Accessories / Associated Devices Affected	
3.	Device Intended Use	

Regulatory Details

Other than India

1.	Device Regulatory Status	Is the device registered globally ☐ Yes ☐ No
		Is the device marketed globally ☐ Yes ☐ No
		If yes provide details :

In India

1.	Device Regulatory Status	Is the device registered in India ☐ Yes ☐ No
		Is the device marketed in India ☐ Yes ☐ No
		If yes provide details :
2.	Manufacturer(s) and Contact Details	
3.	Product License Holder / Local Authorized Representative Name & Address	
4.	Importer(s) / Distributor(s) and Contact Details	

Impacted Device Information

1.	Model Number	
2.	Catalogue Number	
3.	Serial Number	
4.	Affected Lot / Batch Number	
5.	UDI Number	
6.	Accessories / Associated Devices Affected	

1.	Number of affected Unit	**Manufactured in India**
		Period : (mm/yyy) to (mm/yyy)
		Imported into India
		Period : (mm/yyy) to (mm/yyy)
		Supplied in India
		Period : (mm/yyy) to (mm/yyy)
		Expected Shipment to India
		Expected Date of Arrival : (mm/yyy)
2.	Number of affected units supplied to each consignee	
3.	FSCA Strategy	
4.	Did the FSCA arise due to an adverse event?	☐ Yes ☐ No
5.	If yes, what is the category of adverse event?	☐ Serious Public Health Threat ☐ Death ☐ Serious Injury ☐ Non-Serious Injury
6.	Did this adverse event occur in India?	☐ Yes ☐ No If Yes then adverse event Ref. No. & Summary :
7.	Evaluation of risk associated with affected device (Health Hazard Evaluation Report)	
8.	Give reason & detail for FSCA (if other than the adverse event)	

For Other than India

1.	Has the FSCA communication been sent to all consignees?	
2.	Date of commencement of FSCA by product owner (dd/mm/yyy)	
3.	Date of commencement of FSCA (if applicable)	
4.	Countries to which FSCA has been reported (if any)	
5.	Proposed date of completion of FSCA (if applicable)	
6.	Summary of root cause analysis	
7.	Summary of Corrective and Preventive Action (CAPA)	

For India

1.	Affected device details	
2.	Has the FSCA communication been sent to all consignees?	☐ Yes, Date Sent : (dd/mm/yyy) ☐ No (dd/mm/yyy) Expected Date to be sent :
3.	Date of commencement of FSCA by product owner (dd/mm/yyy)	
4.	Date of commencement of FSCA in India (if applicable)	
5.	Countries to which FSCA has been reported (if any)	
6.	Proposed date of completion of FSCA (if applicable)	

7.	Summary of root cause analysis	
8.	Summary of Corrective and Preventive Action (CAPA)	

1.	Type of change (software change, design change, labelling)	
2.	For software change, have any feature not related to FSCA incorporates	☐ Yes ☐ No If Yes then provide details :

I attested that the information submitted is true and accurate and that I am authorized to submit this form in behalf of company.

Signature : ....

Name of reporting person : ....

Date of Notification : ....

PHARMACOVIGILANCE OF
AYURVEDA, SIDDHA, UNANI and HOMOEOPATHY (ASU & H) DRUGS

Reporting Form for Suspected Adverse Reactions

Note:

i.   Personal information of the consumers / patients / ADR reporter's will be kept confidential.
ii. All suspected reactions are to be reported with relevant details.
iii. All completed forms are to be submitted to the program coordinator of nearby centre.

	A / U / S / H
Code	Ay-NIA/Code of Peripheral Centre/ADR Number/Year
	Ay-IPGT/Code of Peripheral Centre/ADR Number/Year
	Un-NIUM/Code of Peripheral Centre/ADR Number/Year
	Si-NIS/Code of Peripheral Centre/ADR Number/Year
	Ho-NIH/Code of Peripheral Centre/ADR Number/Year

1. Patient / consumer identification (please complete or tick boxes below as appropriate)

Name		Patient Record Number
Place of Birth	IPD / OPD	(PRN)
Address Village / Town Post / Via District / State		Age: Sex: Male / Female
Diagnosis:	Constitution and Temperament:	

2. Description of the suspected Adverse Reactions

Date and time of initial observation	
Description of reaction	

3. Whether the patient is suffering with any chronic disorders?

Hepatic   Renal   Cardiac   Diabetes   Any Others

4. Addictions, if any? If yes, please specify:

5. H/O previous allergies / Drug reactions, if any: If yes, please specify:

6. List of all ASU & H drugs used by the patient during the period of one month:

Name of the drug	Manufacturer / Batch no.	Dose	Form / Route of administration	Date of Starting	Date of Stopped / Continued	Reason for use	Any unwanted occurrences

7. **List of other drugs used by the patient during the period of one month:**

Name of the drug	Manufacturer / Batch no.	Dose	Form / Route of administration	Date of		Reason for use	Any unwanted occurrences
				Starting	Stopped / Continued		

8. **Details of the drug suspected to cause ADR:**

    a. Name of the drug:

    b. Manufacturing date and Expiry date (if available):

    c. Remaining pack / label (if available):

    d. Consumed orally along with (water / milk / honey / or any other)

    e. Whether any dietary precautions have been prescribed?
       If yes, please specify :

    f. Whether the drug is consumed under medical supervision or used as self medication.

    g. Any other relevant information associated with drug use:

9. **Management provided / taken for suspected adverse reaction**

10. **Please indicate outcome of the suspected adverse reaction (tick appropriate)**

Recovered:	Not recovered:	Unknown:	Fatal:	If Fatal Date of death:
Severe: Yes / No.	Reaction abated after drug stopped or dose reduced:			
	Reaction reappeared after re administration of drug:			
Was the patient admitted to hospital? If yes, give name and address of hospital				

11. Any abnormal findings of relevant laboratory investigations related to the episode done pre and post episode of ADR:

12. Particulars of ADR Reporter:

Please tick: Patient / Attendant / Nurse / Doctor / Pharmacist / Health worker / Drug Manufacturer / Any others (please specify)
Name:
Address:
Telephone / E - mail:

Signature of the reporter: **Date:**

Please send the completed form to: The centre from where the form is received or to
The Coordinator, National Pharmacovigilance Centre
All India Institute of Ayurveda, Sarita Vihar,
New Delhi - 110 076
Email: pharmacovigilanceayush@gmail.com

The ADR Probability Scale
(Program Coordinator has to fill this scale)

	Questions	Yes	No	Don't Know
1	Are there previous conclusive reports on the reactions?	+1	0	0
2	Did the ADR appear after the suspected drug was administered?	+2	-1	0
3	Did the ADR improve when the drug was discontinued a specific antagonist was administered ?	+1	0	0
4	Did the adverse reaction reappear when the drug was re-administered?	+2	-1	0
5	Are there alternatives causes that could solely have caused the ADR?	-1	+2	0
6	Was the drug detected in the blood (or other fluids) in a concentration known to be toxic?	+1	0	0
7	Was the reaction more severe when the dose was increased, or less severe when the dose was decreased?	+1	0	0
8	Did the patient have a similar reaction to the same or similar drugs in any previous exposure?	+1	0	0
9	Was the adverse event confirmed by objective evidence?	+1	0	0
	Total Score			

Score: > 9 = Certain;   5-8 = Probable;   1-4 = Possible;   0 = Unlikely

Signature
Program Coordinator

Appendix (j)

CIOMS FORM

SUSPECT ADVERSE REACTION REPORT

I. REACTION INFORMATION

1. PATIENT INITIALS (first, last)	1a. COUNTRY	2. DATE OF BIRTH			2a. AGE Years	3. SEX	4-6 REACTION ONSET			8-12 CHECK ALL APPROPRIATE TO ADVERSE REACTION
		Day	Month	Year			Day	Month	Year	

7 + 13 DESCRIBE REACTION(S) (including relevant tests/lab data)

8-12 CHECK ALL APPROPRIATE TO ADVERSE REACTION

☐ PATIENT DIED

☐ INVOLVED OR PROLONGED INPATIENT HOSPITALISATION

☐ INVOLVED PERSISTENCE OR SIGNIFICANT DISABILITY OR INCAPACITY

☐ LIFE THREATENING

II. SUSPECT DRUG(S) INFORMATION

14. SUSPECT DRUG(S) (include generic name)

20 DID REACTION ABATE AFTER STOPPING DRUG? ☐ YES ☐ NO ☐ NA

15. DAILY DOSE(S)

16. ROUTE(S) OF ADMINISTRATION

21. DID REACTION REAPPEAR AFTER REINTRO-DUCTION? ☐ YES ☐ NO ☐ NA

17. INDICATION(S) FOR USE

18. THERAPY DATES (from/to)

19. THERAPY DURATION

III. CONCOMITANT DRUG(S) AND HISTORY

22. CONCOMITANT DRUG(S) AND DATES OF ADMINISTRATION (exclude those used to treat reaction)

23. OTHER RELEVANT HISTORY (e.g. diagnostics, allergics, pregnancy with last month of period, etc.)

IV. MANUFACTURER INFORMATION

24a. NAME AND ADDRESS OF MANUFACTURER

24b. MFR CONTROL NO.

24c. DATE RECEIVED BY MANUFACTURER

24d. REPORT SOURCE ☐ STUDY ☐ LITERATURE ☐ HEALTH PROFESSIONAL

DATE OF THIS REPORT

25a. REPORT TYPE ☐ INITIAL ☐ FOLLOWUP

7. List of other drugs used by the patient during the period of one month:

Name of the drug	Manufacturer / Batch no.	Dose	Form / Route of administration	Date of		Reason for use	Any unwanted occurrences
				Starting	Stopped / Continued		

8. Details of the drug suspected to cause ADR:

   a. Name of the drug:
   b. Manufacturing date and Expiry date (if available):
   c. Remaining pack / label (if available):
   d. Consumed orally along with (water / milk / honey / or any other)
   e. Whether any dietary precautions have been prescribed?
      If yes, please specify :

   f. Whether the drug is consumed under medical supervision or used as self medication.
   g. Any other relevant information associated with drug use:

9. Management provided / taken for suspected adverse reaction

10. Please indicate outcome of the suspected adverse reaction (tick appropriate)

Recovered:	Not recovered:	Unknown:	Fatal:	If Fatal Date of death:
Severe: Yes / No.	Reaction abated after drug stopped or dose reduced:			
	Reaction reappeared after re administration of drug:			
Was the patient admitted to hospital? If yes, give name and address of hospital				

11. Any abnormal findings of relevant laboratory investigations related to the episode done pre and post episode of ADR:

12. Particulars of ADR Reporter:

Please tick:	Patient / Attendant / Nurse / Doctor / Pharmacist / Health worker / Drug Manufacturer / Any others (please specify)
Name:	
Address:	
Telephone / E - mail:	

Signature of the reporter: **Date:**

Please send the completed form to: The centre from where the form is received or to
The Coordinator, National Pharmacovigilance Centre
All India Institute of Ayurveda, Sarita Vihar,
New Delhi - 110 076
Email: pharmacovigilanceayush@gmail.com

The ADR Probability Scale
(Program Coordinator has to fill this scale)

	Questions	Yes	No	Don't Know
1	Are there previous conclusive reports on the reactions?	+1	0	0
2	Did the ADR appear after the suspected drug was administered?	+2	-1	0
3	Did the ADR improve when the drug was discontinued a specific antagonist was administered ?	+1	0	0
4	Did the adverse reaction reappear when the drug was re-administered?	+2	-1	0
5	Are there alternatives causes that could solely have caused the ADR?	-1	+2	0
6	Was the drug detected in the blood (or other fluids) in a concentration known to be toxic?	+1	0	0
7	Was the reaction more severe when the dose was increased, or less severe when the dose was decreased?	+1	0	0
8	Did the patient have a similar reaction to the same or similar drugs in any previous exposure?	+1	0	0
9	Was the adverse event confirmed by objective evidence?	+1	0	0
	Total Score			

Score: > 9 = Certain;   5-8 = Probable;   1-4 = Possible;   0 = Unlikely

Signature
Program Coordinator

Appendix (k)

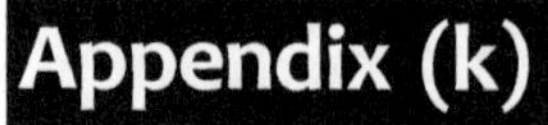

YellowCard
COMMISSION ON HUMAN MEDICINES (CHM)

It's easy to report online at
www.mhra.gov.uk/yellowcard

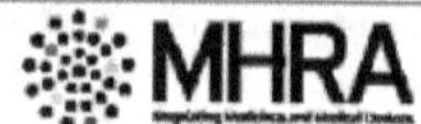

REPORT OF SUSPECTED ADVERSE DRUG REACTIONS

If you suspect an adverse reaction may be related to one or more drugs/vaccines/complementary remedies, please complete this Yellow Card. See 'Adverse reactions to drugs' section in the British National Formulary (BNF) or www.mhra.gov.uk/yellowcard for guidance. Do not be put off reporting because some details are not known.

PATIENT DETAILS   Patient Initials:__________   Sex: M / F   Is the patient pregnant? Y / N   Ethnicity:__________

Age (at time of reaction):________   Weight (kg):________   Identification number (e.g. Practice or Hospital Ref):__________

SUSPECTED DRUG(S)/VACCINE(S)

Drug/Vaccine (Brand if known)	Batch	Route	Dosage	Date started	Date stopped	Prescribed for

SUSPECTED REACTION(S)

Please describe the reaction(s) and any treatment given. (Please attach additional pages if necessary):

Outcome
Recovered ☐
Recovering ☐
Continuing ☐
Other ☐

Date reaction(s) started:__________   Date reaction(s) stopped:__________

Do you consider the reactions to be serious?   Yes / No

If yes, please indicate why the reaction is considered to be serious (please tick all that apply):

☐ Patient died due to reaction   ☐ Involved or prolonged inpatient hospitalisation

☐ Life threatening   ☐ Involved persistent or significant disability or incapacity

☐ Congenital abnormality   Medically significant; please give details:__________

If the reactions were not serious according to the categories above, how bad was the suspected reaction?

☐ Mild   ☐ Unpleasant, but did not affect everyday activities   ☐ Bad enough to affect everyday activities

OTHER DRUG(S) (including self-medication and complementary remedies)

Did the patient take any other medicines/vaccines/complementary remedies in the last 3 months prior to the reaction? Yes / No
If yes, please give the following information if known:

Drug/Vaccine (Brand if known)	Batch	Route	Dosage	Date started	Date stopped	Prescribed for

Additional relevant information e.g. medical history, test results, known allergies, rechallenge (if performed). For reactions relating to use of a medicine during pregnancy please state all other drugs taken during pregnancy, the last menstrual period, information on previous pregnancies, ultrasound scans, any delivery complications, birth defects or developmental concerns.

Please list any medicines obtained from the internet:

REPORTER DETAILS	**CLINICIAN (if not the reporter)**
Name and Professional Address:__________	Name and Professional Address:__________
Postcode:________ Tel No:________	Postcode:________ Tel No:________
Email:__________	Email:__________
Speciality:__________	Speciality:__________
Signature:________ Date:________	Date:__________

Information on adverse drug reactions received by the MHRA can be downloaded at www.mhra.gov.uk/daps
Stay up-to-date on the latest advice for the safe use of medicines with our monthly bulletin *Drug Safety Update* at
www.mhra.gov.uk/drugsafetyupdate

Please attach additional pages if necessary. Send to: FREEPOST YELLOW CARD (no other address details required)

SECOND FOLD HERE

GUIDELINES FOR YELLOW CARD REPORTING

Please use the Yellow Card Scheme to tell us about:

- **All** suspected adverse drug reactions **for new medicines** - identified by the black triangle ▼ symbol
- **All** suspected adverse drug reactions occurring **in children**, even if a medicine has been used off-label
- **All serious*** suspected adverse drug reactions for established vaccines and medicines, including unlicensed medicines, herbal remedies, and medicines used off-label
- **All medication errors** that **result in an adverse reaction**

*Reactions which are fatal, life-threatening, a congenital abnormality, disabling or incapacitating, result in or prolong hospitalisation, or medically significant are considered serious.

If you are unsure, please report anyway

For more information:

- Contact the Yellow Card Information Service on Freephone 0800 731 6789
- Visit the Yellow Card website – **www.mhra.gov.uk/yellowcard**

FIRST FOLD HERE

Appendix (I)

Reset Form

U.S. Department of Health and Human Services

MEDWATCH

The FDA Safety Information and
Adverse Event Reporting Program

For VOLUNTARY reporting of
adverse events, product problems and
product use errors

Page 1 of 3

Form Approved: OMB No. 0910-0291. Expires: 6/30/2015
See PRA statement on reverse.

FDA USE ONLY

Triage unit
sequence #

A. PATIENT INFORMATION

1. Patient Identifier	2. Age at Time of Event or Date of Birth:	3. Sex	4. Weight
In confidence		☐ Female ☐ Male	___ lb or ___ kg

B. ADVERSE EVENT, PRODUCT PROBLEM OR ERROR

Check all that apply:

1. ☐ Adverse Event   ☐ Product Problem (e.g., defects/malfunctions)
   ☐ Product Use Error   ☐ Problem with Different Manufacturer of Same Medicine

2. Outcomes Attributed to Adverse Event
   (Check all that apply)
   ☐ Death: _______ (mm/dd/yyyy)
   ☐ Life-threatening
   ☐ Hospitalization - initial or prolonged
   ☐ Required Intervention to Prevent Permanent Impairment/Damage (Devices)
   ☐ Disability or Permanent Damage
   ☐ Congenital Anomaly/Birth Defect
   ☐ Other Serious (Important Medical Events)

3. Date of Event (mm/dd/yyyy) | 4. Date of this Report (mm/dd/yyyy)

5. Describe Event, Problem or Product Use Error

(Continue on page 3)

6. Relevant Tests/Laboratory Data, Including Dates

(Continue on page 3)

7. Other Relevant History, Including Preexisting Medical Conditions (e.g., allergies, race, pregnancy, smoking and alcohol use, liver/kidney problems, etc.)

(Continue on page 3)

C. PRODUCT AVAILABILITY

Product Available for Evaluation? (Do not send product to FDA)

☐ Yes   ☐ No   ☐ Returned to Manufacturer on: _______ (mm/dd/yyyy)

D. SUSPECT PRODUCT(S)

1. Name, Strength, Manufacturer (from product label)
   #1 Name:
      Strength:
      Manufacturer:
   #2 Name:
      Strength:
      Manufacturer:

2. Dose or Amount | Frequency | Route
   #1
   #2

3. Dates of Use (if unknown, give duration) from/to (or best estimate)
   #1
   #2

4. Diagnosis or Reason for Use (Indication)
   #1
   #2

5. Event Abated After Use Stopped or Dose Reduced?
   #1 ☐ Yes ☐ No ☐ Doesn't Apply
   #2 ☐ Yes ☐ No ☐ Doesn't Apply

6. Event Reappeared After Reintroduction?
   #1 ☐ Yes ☐ No ☐ Doesn't Apply
   #2 ☐ Yes ☐ No ☐ Doesn't Apply

6. Lot # | 7. Expiration Date
   #1   #1
   #2   #2

9. NDC # or Unique ID

E. SUSPECT MEDICAL DEVICE

1. Brand Name

2. Common Device Name | 2b. Procode

3. Manufacturer Name, City and State

4. Model # | Lot # | 5. Operator of Device
   Catalog # | Expiration Date (mm/dd/yyyy)   ☐ Health Professional
   Serial # | Unique Identifier (UDI) #   ☐ Lay User/Patient   ☐ Other:

6. If Implanted, Give Date (mm/dd/yyyy) | 7. If Explanted, Give Date (mm/dd/yyyy)

8. Is this a Single-use Device that was Reprocessed and Reused on a Patient?
   ☐ Yes ☐ No

9. If Yes to Item No. 8, Enter Name and Address of Reprocessor

F. OTHER (CONCOMITANT) MEDICAL PRODUCTS

Product names and therapy dates (exclude treatment of event)

(Continue on page 3)

G. REPORTER (See confidentiality section on back)

1. Name and Address
   Name:
   Address:
   City: State: ZIP:
   Phone #:   E-mail:

2. Health Professional? | 3. Occupation | 4. Also Reported to:
   ☐ Yes ☐ No   ☐ Manufacturer
                                                    ☐ User Facility
5. If you do NOT want your identity disclosed   ☐ Distributor/Importer
   to the manufacturer, place an "X" in this box: ☐

PLEASE TYPE OR USE BLACK INK

FORM FDA 3500 (2/13)   Submission of a report does not constitute an admission that medical personnel or the product caused or contributed to the event.

ADVICE ABOUT VOLUNTARY REPORTING
Detailed instructions available at: http://www.fda.gov/medwatch/report/consumer/instruct.htm

Report adverse events, product problems or product use errors with:
- Medications *(drugs or biologics)*
- Medical devices *(including in-vitro diagnostics)*
- Combination products *(medication & medical devices)*
- Human cells, tissues, and cellular and tissue-based products
- Special nutritional products *(dietary supplements, medical foods, infant formulas)*
- Cosmetics
- Food *(including beverages and ingredients added to foods)*

Report product problems - quality, performance or safety concerns such as:
- Suspected counterfeit product
- Suspected contamination
- Questionable stability
- Defective components
- Poor packaging or labeling
- Therapeutic failures (product didn't work)

Report SERIOUS adverse events. An event is serious when the patient outcome is:
- Death
- Life-threatening
- Hospitalization - initial or prolonged
- Disability or permanent damage
- Congenital anomaly/birth defect
- Required intervention to prevent permanent impairment or damage (devices)
- Other serious (important medical events)

Report even if:
- You're not certain the product caused the event
- You don't have all the details

How to report:
- Just fill in the sections that apply to your report
- Use section D for all products except medical devices
- Attach additional pages if needed
- Use a separate form for each patient
- Report either to FDA or the manufacturer *(or both)*

Other methods of reporting:
- 1-800-FDA-0178 - To FAX report
- 1-800-FDA-1088 - To report by phone
- www.fda.gov/medwatch/report.htm - To report online

If your report involves a serious adverse event with a device and it occurred in a facility outside a doctor's office, that facility may be legally required to report to FDA and/or the manufacturer. Please notify the person in that facility who would handle such reporting.

If your report involves a serious adverse event with a vaccine, call 1-800-822-7967 to report.

Confidentiality: The patient's identity is held in strict confidence by FDA and protected to the fullest extent of the law. FDA will not disclose the reporter's identity in response to a request from the public, pursuant to the Freedom of Information Act. The reporter's identity, including the identity of a self-reporter, may be shared with the manufacturer unless requested otherwise.

The information in this box applies only to requirements of the Paperwork Reduction Act of 1995

The burden time for this collection of information has been estimated to average 36 minutes per response, including the time to review instructions, search existing data sources, gather and maintain the data needed, and complete and review the collection of information. Send comments regarding this burden estimate or any other aspect of this collection of information, including suggestions for reducing this burden to:

*Department of Health and Human Services
Food and Drug Administration
Office of Chief Information Officer
Paperwork Reduction Act (PRA) Staff
PRAStaff@fda.hhs.gov*

*Please DO NOT
RETURN this form
to the PRA Staff e-mail
to the left.*

*OMB statement:
"An agency may not conduct or sponsor, and a person is not required to respond to, a collection of information unless it displays a currently valid OMB control number."*

U.S. DEPARTMENT OF HEALTH AND HUMAN SERVICES
Food and Drug Administration

FORM FDA 3500 (2/13) (Back)   Please Use Address Provided Below -- Fold in Thirds, Tape and Mail

---

**DEPARTMENT OF
HEALTH & HUMAN SERVICES**

Public Health Service
Food and Drug Administration
Rockville, MD 20857

Official Business
Penalty for Private Use $300

NO POSTAGE
NECESSARY
IF MAILED
IN THE
UNITED STATES
OR APO/FPO

BUSINESS REPLY MAIL
FIRST CLASS MAIL PERMIT NO. 946 ROCKVILLE MD

POSTAGE WILL BE PAID BY FOOD AND DRUG ADMINISTRATION

MEDWATCH
The FDA Safety Information and Adverse Event Reporting Program
Food and Drug Administration
5600 Fishers Lane
Rockville, MD 20852-9787

B.5. Describe Event or Problem *(continued)*

Back to Form

B.6. Relevant Tests/Laboratory Data, Including Dates *(continued)*

Back to Form

B.7. Other Relevant History, Including Preexisting Medical Conditions *(e.g., allergies, race, pregnancy, smoking and alcohol use, hepatic/renal dysfunction, etc.) (continued)*

Back to Form

F. Concomitant Medical Products and Therapy Dates *(Exclude treatment of event) (continued)*

Back to Form

Appendix (m)

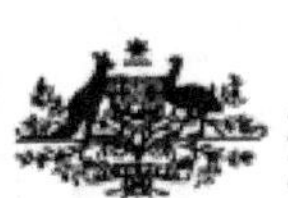

Australian Government

Department of Health
Therapeutic Goods Administration

TGA use only

Report of suspected adverse reaction to medicines or vaccines

See statement about the collection and use of personal information overleaf, and please attach any additional data to this form

Patient initials or medical record number:	Sex: M ☐ F ☐	Date of birth or age:
	Weight (kg):	

Suspected medicine(s)/vaccine(s)

Medicine/vaccine (please use trade names; include batch number and AUST R or AUST L number if known)	**Dosage** (Dose number for vaccines eg 1ˢᵗ DTP)	Date begun	Date stopped	Reason for use

Other medicine(s)/vaccine(s) taken at the time of the reaction

Medicine/vaccine	**Dosage**	Date begun	Date stopped	Reason for use

Reaction(s):   Date of onset of reaction (for vaccines time after administration):   /   /

Describe: (please provide as much detail as possible and include any results of relevant laboratory data and other investigations)

Seriousness: Life threatening ☐   Hospitalised ☐   Required a visit to doctor ☐

Treatment of reaction:

Outcome: Recovered ☐ ▶ Date: /   /   Not yet recovered ☐   Fatal ☐ ▶ Date: /   /   Unknown ☐

Sequelae?   No ☐   Yes ☐ ▶ Describe:

Reporting: Doctor ☐   Pharmacist ☐   Other ☐   Contact details (email or phone)

Name:

Address:

Signature:

Postcode: Date: /   /

Thank you for taking the time to complete this form   PTO

Report of suspected reaction to medicines or vaccines ("Blue card")

Fold here first (Please do not use staples on this form)

Phone: 1800 044 114   www.tga.gov.au/reporting-problems   Email: adr.reports@tga.gov.au   Fax: 02 6232 8392

What to report
You do not need to be certain, just suspicious!

Any information related to the reporter and patient identifiers is kept strictly confidential.

Adverse drug reaction reports should be submitted for prescription medicines, vaccines, over-the-counter medicines (medicines purchased without a prescription), and complementary medicines (herbal medicines, naturopathic and/or homoeopathic medicines, and nutritional supplements such as vitamins and minerals). Please include timing of reactions relative to medicine administration where relevant.

The TGA particularly requests reports of:

- All suspected reactions to new medicines and vaccines
- All suspected drug interactions
- Unexpected reactions, that is not consistent with product information or labelling
- Serious reactions which are suspected of significantly affecting a patient's management, including reactions suspected of causing death, danger to life, admission to hospital, prolongation of hospitalisation, absence from productive activity, increased investigational or treatment costs, and birth defects.

Fold here second

D1073 February 2015

(Event checklist)

Note: Y: Yes; N: No; UK: Unknown; NA: Not applicable

I. Is there strong evidence for other causes?	Y	N	UK	NA	Remarks
Does a clinical examination, or laboratory tests on the patient, confirm another cause?	☐	☐	☐	☐	
II. Is there a known causal association with the vaccine or vaccination?					
Vaccine product(s)					
Is there evidence in the literature that this vaccine(s) may cause the reported event even if administered correctly?	☐	☐	☐	☐	
Did a specific test demonstrate the causal role of the vaccine or any of the ingredients?	☐	☐	☐	☐	
Immunization error					
Was there an error in prescribing or non-adherence to recommendations for use of the vaccine (use beyond the expiry date, wrong recipient, etc.)?	☐	☐	☐	☐	
Was the vaccine (or any of its ingredients) administered unsterile?	☐	☐	☐	☐	
Was the vaccine's physical condition (colour, turbidity, presence of foreign substances) abnormal at the time of administration?	☐	☐	☐	☐	
Was there an error in vaccine constitution/preparation by the vaccinator (wrong product, wrong diluent, improper mixing, improper syringe filling)?	☐	☐	☐	☐	
Was there an error in vaccine handling (a break in the cold chain during transport, storage and/or immunization session)?	☐	☐	☐	☐	
Was the vaccine administered incorrectly (wrong dose, site or route of administration; wrong needle size)?	☐	☐	☐	☐	
Immunization anxiety					
Could the event have been caused by anxiety about the immunization (vasovagal, hyperventilation or stress-related disorder)?	☐	☐	☐	☐	
II (time). If "Yes" to any question in II, was the event within the time window of increased risk?					
Did the event occur within an appropriate time window after vaccine administration?	☐	☐	☐	☐	
III. Is there strong evidence against a causal association?					
Is there strong evidence against a causal association?	☐	☐	☐	☐	
IV. Other qualifying factors for classification					
Could the event occur independently of vaccination (background rate)?	☐	☐	☐	☐	
Could the event be a manifestation of another health condition?	☐	☐	☐	☐	
Did a comparable event occur after a previous dose of a similar vaccine?	☐	☐	☐	☐	
Was there exposure to a potential risk factor or toxin prior to the event?	☐	☐	☐	☐	
Was there acute illness prior to the event?	☐	☐	☐	☐	
Did the event occur in the past independently of vaccination?	☐	☐	☐	☐	
Was the patient taking any medication prior to vaccination?	☐	☐	☐	☐	
Is there a biological plausibility that the vaccine could cause the event?	☐	☐	☐	☐	

Glossary

Absolute Risk: Risk in a population of exposed persons. Absolute risk can be measured in over time or at a given time.

Adverse (Drug) Event: Any untoward medical occurrence that may present during treatment with a pharmaceutical product which does not necessarily have a causal relationship with the treatment. [An event is any new clinical experience that occurs after commencing treatment with a medicine regardless of its severity or seriousness and without judgement on its causality. Favourable events may be recorded as an indication of an unexpected therapeutic effect. ADR in a patient is an adverse outcome that is attributed to a suspected action of a drug while the Adverse Event is an adverse outcome that occurs after the use of a drug, *but which may or may not be linked to use of the drug*. All ADRs are Adverse (Drug) Events but the reverse is not true. All Adverse (Drug) Events are not necessarily ADRs]. Example of adverse drug event: Heart arrhythmia from discontinuing atenolol (whether or not is an error); Example of adverse drug reaction: skin rashes from nevirapine.

Adverse Drug Reaction (ADR): A response to a medicine that is noxious and unintended and occurs at doses normally used in man for prophylaxis, diagnosis, or therapy of disease, or for the modification of physiological function. The WHO definition excludes well known side effects. Side effects are usually noxious, unintended but expected in usual dose. But the ADR is not expected. This ADR definition does not include intentional or accidental poisoning or drug abuse too. [Adverse Drug Reaction and Adverse Drug Event are often used interchangeably. Adverse reaction refers to the patient point of view while adverse effect applies to the drug]. An adverse reaction, contrary to the adverse event, is characterised by the suspicion of a causal relationship between the drug and occurrence: judged possibly by reporting or reviewing by health professional. An ADR is always an ADE but ADE need not be ADR. ADE may be due to overdose caused by dispensing error.

Adverse Events Following Immunization (AEFI): Medical Incident that takes place after an immunization causes concern and is believed to have caused by immunization.

Attributable Risk: Difference between the risk in an exposed population (absolute risk) and the risk in an unexposed population. This is also known as excess risk.

Audit Finding(s): Results of the evaluation of the collected evidence against prefixed criteria.

Audit Plan: Description of activities and arrangement for an assessment.

Audit Programme: Set of one or more audits planned for a specific timeframe and for a specific purpose.

Audit Recommendation: Activities that the management might consider to rectify conditions that have gone away and to mitigate weaknesses in systems of management control. Audit recommendations should be positive and as specific as possible. They should also identify who is to act on them.

Audit: A systematic, disciplined, independent and documented process for obtaining evidence and evaluating it objectively to determine the extent of compliance to policies, procedures and requirements.

Benefit –Risk Analysis: Examination of the favourable and unfavourable results for undertaking a specific course of action.

Benefit: An estimated gain for an individual or population.

Bioethics: Ethical principles of biomedical research in human beings.

Causality Assessment: The evaluation of likelihood that a medicine was the causative agent of an observed adverse event.

Clinical Trial: Human experimentations for assessing the safety and efficacy of a medicinal product.

Cohort Event Monitoring: A prospective observational study of adverse events associated with one or more medicines.

Dechallenge: The withdrawal of the drug following suspected adverse drug reaction.

Effectiveness: The ability of the medicine to produce the desired beneficial effect in actual use.

Efficacy: The ability of the drug to produce the intended effects under ideal conditions of use.

Electronic Health Record Mining: Scanning of electronic health record for detecting desired information.

Individual Case Safety Report: A suspected adverse drug reaction report that occurred in an individual patient.

Informed Consent: Providing acceptance for participating in the research with full knowledge and understanding the risk and benefit.

Naranjo Probability Scale: A tool used to establish a relationship between an adverse event and the suspected drug.

Periodic Adverse Drug Experience Report [PADER]/Periodic Adverse Experience Report (PAER): Periodically developed safety data for submission to US FDA. These are previous format for submitting PSUR, now replaced with PBRER.

Periodic Benefit Risk Evaluation Report (PBRER): US FDA requirement to submit safety and benefit report at predetermined interval for a marketed product. This is a new format for submitting PSUR (now the term is changed).

Periodic Safety Update Report [PSUR]: A document periodically developed containing comprehensive worldwide safety data of a marketed product.

Pharmacogenetics: The use of genetic markers to maximise the safety and/or efficacy of drugs.

Pharmacovigilance: The science and activities relating to the detection, assessment, understanding and prevention of adverse effects or any other drug related problem.

Polypharmacy: The concomitant use of more than one drug.

Quality Adherence: Carrying out tasks and responsibilities in accordance with quality requirements.

Quality Assurance: The planned and systematic activities designed and carried out in a system so that the quality requirement for a programme or system is ensured.

Quality Control: Part of quality management focussed on fulfilling quality requirements like characteristics of a product, process or system.

Quality Improvements: Correcting and improving the structures and processes where necessary. This applies for the purpose of fulfilling quality requirements.

Quality of a Pharmacovigilance System: All characteristics of the pharmacovigilance system which are considered to be in consistent to the objectives of pharmacovigilance.

Quality Planning: Establishing structures and planning of integrated and consistent processes to fulfil quality requirements.

Quality Requirements: Those characteristics of a system likely to produce the desired outcome.

Quality System of a Pharmacovigilance System: The organisational structure, responsibilities, procedures and resources of the pharmacovigilance system responsible for quality outcomes.

Rechallenge: The drug is given again to the patient after withdrawal (following suspected adverse drug reaction) on complete recovery of ADR symptoms.

Record Linkage: Methods of assembling information contained in two or more records.

Relative Risk: The ratio of the risk in an exposed population (absolute risk) and the risk in an unexposed population.

Risk: The probability of harm being caused.

Serious Adverse Events (or, Serious Adverse Drug Reaction): A serious adverse event or reaction is any untoward medical occurrence that at any dose: results in death, hospitalization or prolongation of hospitalization, persistent or significant disability or incapacity, life threatening, a congenital anomaly or birth defect. [The two terminologies serious and severe often cause confusion and are not synonymous. They cannot be used interchangeably. Severe describes the intensity (severity) of an event and the event may be minor medical significance (severe headache). On the other hand, seriousness (not severity) refers the outcome of the event on the patient].

Side Effect: Any unintended effect of a medicine occurring at doses normally used in human which is related to pharmacological properties of the medicine. But it could be beneficial too.

Signal: Reported information on a possible causal relationship between an adverse event and a drug, the relationship being unknown or incompletexy documented previously. Usually more than a single report is necessary to generate a signal, depending on the seriousness of the event and the quality of information.

Spontaneous Report: Unsolicited communication by healthcare professionals or consumers that describes one or more ADRs in a patient who was given one or more medicinal products and that does not derive from a study or any organized data collection scheme.

VigiAccess: Open access to WHO database of suspected adverse drug reactions.

VigiBase: WHO database of individual case safety report.

VigiFlow: Spontaneous reporting data entry and analytical tool for WHO database.

VigiLyze: Powerful search and analysis tool that provide access to WHO database and instantly provides data in graph and table format.

VigiMed: Forum that provides access to safety concern in other countries [WHO Programme].

VigiMine: Data Mining tool as a part of VigiSearch.

VigiSearch: Search tool for searching VigiBase database.

Websites of Interest and Some Important References

1. https://cdsco.gov.in/opencms/opencms/en/Home/

2. http://www.pvpi.in/

3. http://www.ich.org/

4. http://www.isoponline.org/

5. http://www.who.int/medicines/areas/quality_safety/safety_efficacy/pharmvigi/en/index.html

6. http://www.who.int/medicines/publications/newsletter/en/

7. http://www.who-pvafrica.org/index.php/pharmacovigilance

8. http://www.who-umc.org/DynPage.aspx?id=105825&mn1=7347&mn2=7259&mn3=7297&mn4=7494

9. https://www.facebook.com/SOPI.India/

10. https://www.pharmacoepi.org/

11. Asian Pharmacoepidemiology Network: http://www.aspennet.asia/

12. Australian Prescriber: http://www.australianprescriber.com/

13. Central Drug Standard Control Organization

14. Council for international Organization of Medical Sciences

15. Current Challenges in Pharmacovigilance: Pragmatic Approaches, Report of CIOMS Working Group V, CIOMS, Geneva, 2001.

16. Guidance for Industry on Pharmacovigilance Requirements for Biological Products, Central Drugs Standard Control Organization, Ministry of Health and Family Welfare, Government of India, 2017.

17. Guru Prasad Mohanta, Textbook on Clinical Research: A Guide for Aspiring Professionals and Professionals, Second Edition, PharmaMed Press, 2017.

18. International Council for Harmonization of Technical Requirements for Pharmaceuticals for Human Use

19. International Society for Pharmacoepidemiology: https://www.pharmacoepi.org/

20. International Society of Pharmacovigilance: https://isoponline.org/

21. Management of Safety Information from Clinical Trials, Report of CIOMS Working Group VI, CIOMS, Geneva, 2005.

22. Patrick Waller, An Introduction to Pharmacovigilance, Wiley – Blackwell, UK, 2010.

23. Pharmacovigilance Guidance Document for Marketing Authorization Holders of Pharmaceutical Products, Indian Pharmacopeia Commission, Government of India, 2018.

24. Pharmacovigilance Toolkit: http://pvtoolkit.org/

25. Raman Sehgal, RajatSethi and Shobha Rani Hiremath, Elements of Pharmacovigilance, Kongposh Publication, New Delhi, 2010.

26. Ronald D. Mann and Elizabeth Andrews (Ed), Pharmacovigilance, Second Edition, John Wiley & Sons Limited, England, 2007.

27. S. K. Gupta (Ed), Textbook of Pharmacovigilance, Jaypee Brothers Medical Publishers (P) Ltd., New Delhi, 2011.

28. Safety of Medicines, World Health Organization, Geneva, 2002.

29. Society of Pharmacovigilance, India.

30. The Importance of Pharmacovigilance, World Health Organization, 2002.

31. The Uppsala Monitoring Centre: http://www.who-umc.org/

32. Uppsala Reports

33. View Point – Part 1, the Uppsala Monitoring Centre, 2002.

34. View Point – Part 2, the Uppsala Monitoring Centre, 2005.

35. WHO Collaborating Centre for Advocacy and Training in Pharmacovigilance:

36. WHO Pharmaceuticals Newsletter

37. WHO Policy Perspectives on Medicines – Pharmacovigilance: ensuring the safe use of medicines, WHO, October 2004.

38. World Health Organization Website.

Index